The Polar
FAT FREE and
FIT FOREVER
Program

∙∙∙

by **Dr. James M. Rippe** *with Karla Dougherty*

FIRESIDE
Rockefeller Center
1230 Avenue of the Americas
New York, New York 10020

Cover design by CIS/Finland
Interior design by Fabia Wargin/Creative Media Applications

Manufactured in the United States of America

10 9 8 7 6 5 4 3 2 1

Library of Congress Cataloging in Publication data

ISBN: 0-671-88881-1

Acknowledgement is made for permission to use or reprint the following:

Rippe, J.M., Ward, A., *The Complete Book of Fitness Walking*, New York: Prentice Hall Press, 1990.
Rippe, J.M., *The Exercise Exchange Program*, New York: Simon & Schuster, 1992.
Rippe, J.M., *Dr. James M. Rippe's Fit for Success: Proven Strategies for Executive Health*, New York: Prentice Hall Press, 1989.
Rippe, J.M., Ward, A., *The Rockport Walking Program*, New York: Fireside Press, 1989.
Rippe, J.M., Southmayd, W., *The Sports Performance Factors*, New York: Perigee Books, 1986.
Copyright ©1993 by The STEP Company. Fitness Stepping™ is a trademark of The STEP Company.

Cover photo credits:

Center photo: Paul Barton/The Stock Market
Bottom right photo: Walter Hodges/ALLSTOCK

TABLE OF CONTENTS

The Polar Program Method

"It's like having your own personal trainer."

— A 40-year-old woman on the Polar Fat Free and Fit Forever Program

A group of people changed their lives this summer.

They didn't win millions in the lottery. They didn't move up the corporate ladder to CEO. They didn't meet the idealized person of their dreams. What they did wasn't wishful thinking. It was real. It was positive and full of hope.

These individuals began to take charge of their bodies, their health and, ultimately, their lives.

They learned how to fight back against a lifetime of being overweight. They learned how to fight back against a lifetime of bad habits. They learned how to fight back against the stubborn fat cells that can prevent long-term weight loss and long-term cardiovascular health.

It began in June, 1993 at our exercise laboratory at the University of Massachussetts Medical Center. We were looking for individuals who wanted to try a new way to lose weight and, as soon as an ad was placed in a local Massachusetts paper, the calls rang off the hook.

The people we ultimately chose ranged in age from 20 to 49. They were all relatively healthy women at least 20 percent overweight. The rules of the game? They were to follow a loosely structured low-fat diet in which only 23 percent of their calories came from fat. They were to walk three to five times a week for a seven-day total of 13 to 15 miles at a fat burning, aerobic intensity.

But here's the difference between this program and all the rest: these individuals were to wear a Polar Heart Rate Monitor each and every time they walked. The Polar Heart Rate Monitor, a lightweight, wireless fitness monitor, showed the individuals when they were exercising in their effective cardiovascular heart rate zone — so that they could improve aerobic performance, lose weight, and burn fat effectively.

The study lasted twelve weeks — and the results were phenomenal. The individuals lost an average of seven and a half pounds — but they lost an average of **eight pounds of body fat** which translated into an impressive decrease of 10 percent in body fat. They also had significant increases in their fitness, which included an eight percent increase in their aerobic stamina—while maintaining 100 percent of their lean muscle tissue. Traditional diets without proper exercise do not provide these fitness and health benefits.

In other words, **these individuals lost weight in body fat without any loss of vital muscle tissue.**

Further, during our present six-month follow-up study, we are finding that these people are continuing to make their healthy lifestyle changes a habit.

It isn't a miracle. All of us know that reducing fat and increasing activity can help stave off the fat cell's cry of "feed me" which leads to a slower metabolism and weight gain. Indeed, as much as we look to "quick fixes," we know that nothing works in the long run except eating fewer calories and doing more. There have been countless studies conducted to substantiate these claims — many of them at our laboratory alone.

The people in our study knew all about fad diets and the reality of real weight loss. They knew how difficult it was to keep on track when it comes to a sensible weight management program — which made their success even more impressive. The miracle is how **easily** these people changed their lives — and how they are continuing to keep it up, despite hectic schedules and the erratic nature of life stress. Even today, they remain highly motivated.

The key to this "miracle?" The Polar Heart Rate Monitor they wore every time they walked. As this study shows, there is clear evidence that the use of a Polar Heart Rate Monitor can directly affect weight management success.

WHY POLAR MAKES A DIFFERENCE

A t first glance, the Polar Heart Rate Monitor looks like a simple wrist watch. But the lightweight strap that is worn around your chest is actually a marvel of electronic technology. It accurately monitors the change in your heart rate as you exercise, and transmits it continuously to the wristwatch receiver. It tells you when to increase or decrease your exercise intensity for maximum and safe results.

Your heart rate is the most important factor for effective weight loss and cardiovascular health. Too low a heart rate and you won't lose weight or receive any aerobic benefit. Too high and you run the risk of injury — or, at the very least, a drop in motivation from fatigue and pain.

But your **target** heart rate zone — or, as we call it, your target weight management zone is the range where your heart is being exercised comfortably and safely without unnecessary strain, to both effectively burn calories and fat and increase your aerobic capacity.

The Polar Heart Rate Monitor takes the confusion out of knowing if you are in your target weight management zone. At a fast glance, it shows you whether or not you are performing at an appropriate aerobic intensity, which can translate into exercise that can:

- Be sustained for longer periods of time
- Build up endurance and strength
- Be more precise than any other measure of improvement
- Maintain a high level of motivation and enjoyment

It's not just a question of peak performance. It's also something intrinsic within the Polar Heart Rate Monitor itself. Suddenly, there is something real, something that is immediately tangible, that is showing you your success. It is guiding you and watching you, and helping you get to the next level of fitness and weight loss.

Just ask the people in our study. The Polar Heart Rate Monitor did what no other weight management program did before: it kept them going strong.

WEIGHT MANAGEMENT: EASIER SAID THAN DONE

In the United States alone, over half of the adult population is overweight and at least 20 percent of them are seriously overweight. Worse, 95 percent of those people who go on diets and lose weight gain their weight back—and more—within two years.

Obviously, there's a problem. Despite the huge amounts of available books, articles, tapes, and programs on weight loss, the figures remain constant.

We have been studying that problem for a decade at the Exercise Physiology Laboratory at the University of Massachusetts Medical Center. We have done studies in aerobic training, strength training, weight loss and cardiovascular health. We have learned that body fat is more important than actual weight — which traditional diets do not take into account. On most diets, people lose important muscle tissue along with their body fat. This proves to be their downfall. Since muscle tissue is metabolic, the more muscle tissue we lose, the more our metabolism slows down — which makes it harder and harder to continue to lose weight.

In our quest at the lab to find a weight management program that reduced body fat while maintaining life-sustaining muscle, we have found that a combination of aerobic exercise along with a low-fat diet works best for long-term success. In further studies at the lab, we found that combining both aerobic exercise and strength training with a low-fat diet not only burns body fat cells while preserving lean muscle tissue — **but it can actually increase the amount of muscle tissue in the body.**

In these studies and others we've conducted over the past ten years, we have consistently relied on the Polar Heart Rate Monitor for precise measurement of our results. Research, of course, demands precision. We need to take highly accurate measurements of heart rate, body fat, aerobic capacity, nutrient content of diets, and more in order to know our findings are correct. The Polar Heart Rate Monitor has always helped us reach that goal.

But what we didn't realize until recently was that the Polar Heart Rate Monitor that gave us our necessary precision was also a highly motivational tool for our subjects. By using their Polar Heart Rate Monitors, many of them found that they gained valuable knowledge and insight into their exercise programs — which kept their motivation high and helped them achieve their weight management goals.

To test this outside interest in the Polar Heart Rate Monitor, we conducted the 12 week Polar study — and the Polar Fat Free and Fit Forever Program was born.

A WINNING COMBINATION

I started studying medicine almost 20 years ago with a simple goal in mind: to help people live the healthiest lives possible by taking charge of their daily habits and lifestyles. Today, this remains my major commitment and, as a cardiologist, author, and director of one of the largest centers of nutrition, exercise, and weight control research in the country, I have been able to help more and more people learn what I have learned: you can make a difference. You can change the way you live.

And, as our 12 week study shows, the Polar Fat Free and Fit Forever Program can help you towards this goal.

POLAR IS THE CHOICE OF PROFESSIONALS

The Polar company was founded in 1977 by Professor Seppo Saynajakangas, an engineer and athlete who was inspired to develop a new method for monitoring heart rate while cross-country skiing. In those days, heart rate was still measured with the finger-tips — a slow and inaccurate process. The professor developed the Polar Heart Rate Monitor's simple structure and brought it to the National Sporting Goods Association in 1985. It was only a matter of time before it was used and endorsed by professional athletes, trainers, and coaches as a precise method for measuring heart rate and performance level.

Indeed, today my research center is only one of many that use the Polar Heart Rate Monitor. The Pritikin Center in California uses them. So does Duke University, the Cooper Clinic, Stanford University, the U.S. Army, the U.S. Air Force, and leading health spas, world class athletes and sports clubs across the country.

Polar is also the choice of Dan Issacson, Hollywood's leading fitness and weight loss trainer. Dan has used Polar Heart Rate Monitors for years to help some of Hollywood's biggest stars get their bodies into great shape. Dan uses Polar Heart Rate Monitors to help Hollywood stars burn off their excess fat and calories, and strengthen their muscle tone and aerobic capacity to look and feel great.

THE SCIENCE OF POLAR

Polar Heart Rate Monitors are so reliable that they are used by the people who **really** need to make accurate assessments. NASA uses Polar Heart Rate Monitors for their astronauts in space shuttle flights to monitor and guide their exercise intensity.

As precise as a physician's electrocardiogram, the Polar Heart Rate Monitor is also used by cardiologists for their cardiac patients because it provides safe, simple, and effective rehabilitation.

Cardiologists, scientists, astronauts, clinical researchers, exercise physiologists, professional trainers, and world class athletes know: monitoring your heart rate is the most scientifically proven method for fitness improvement, fat burning, and long-term weight management. The Polar Heart Rate Monitor is the speedometer for your body. It tells you when to work harder and when to ease off.

POLAR IS FOR EVERYONE

But, as you will see as you read this book, Polar Heart Rate Monitors are for everyone — not just celebrities or astronauts, athletes or fitness trainers. Old, young, fit or "couch potato" alike — all can benefit from the Polar Fat Free and Fit Forever Program.

Like the people in our study, you can use your Polar Heart Rate Monitor and the Polar Precision Weight Management Program to achieve long-term weight management and cardiovascular health. You will find that it is adaptable for different ages, fitness improvement, even life changes such as pregnancy. It can be used for all forms of exercise — from walking and running to weight training and step aerobic class. Even swimmers can successfully use the Polar Fat Free and Fit Forever Program to:

- Burn fat
- Tone and strengthen your body
- Reduce stress
- Promote higher energy

READY, SET GO!

This book will show you how to do it: lose body fat and keep those fat cells quiet once and for all. It will show you how to make more of your lean muscle tissue and keep metabolism high. It will help you find your own unique Polar Fat Free and Fit Forever recipe — to help you lose weight and keep it off.

To that end, we start the book by disclosing the myths about obesity, the "tall tales" that have stopped you from understanding how and why to lose weight successfully. We then take you through a series of self-tests to find your Polar Fat Free and Fit Forever "niche" — where you will find your own individual recipe for low-fat living and effective exercise. We even guide you through your first week of the program — and beyond.

And, throughout these pages, you'll also find hints and suggestions to keep motivation strong and spirits high.

Are you ready?

Let's go.....

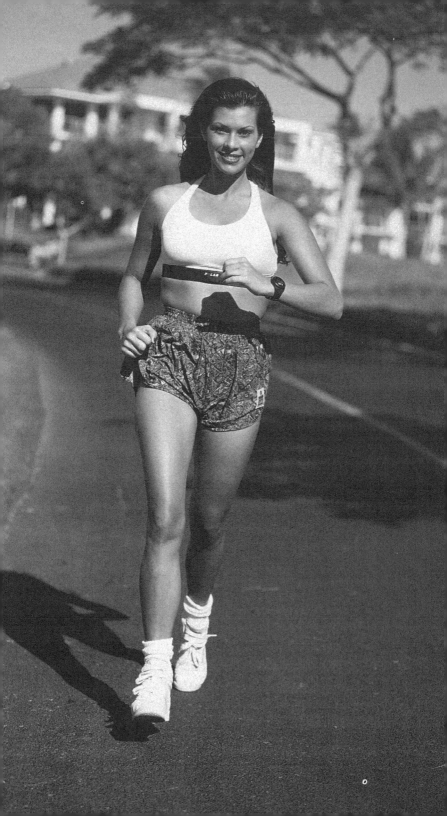

The Real Facts

"I knew I needed to exercise more to lose weight,

About Fat,

but I didn't really understand why — or how to do it right.

Exercise, and

Polar makes it all clear for me. Plus it keeps me going."

Your Health

— A 38-year-old executive on the Polar Fat Free and Fit Forever Program

Before you can solve algebraic equations, you need to learn basic math. Before you can paint with oils, you need to learn the fundamentals of color. Similarly, before you can successfully embark on any weight management program, you have to understand the underlying mechanics behind the caloric regulation and the exercise regime. You have to understand how your program effectively influences long-term weight loss, physical fitness, and health.

THE "WHYS" BEHIND THE "WHATS"

A weight management program is more than a step-by-step, "by the book" routine. Following directions by rote without a deeper understanding of **the why** keeps things on the surface — which makes you vulnerable to getting off track whenever a diversion or stressful situation comes your way. For a lifelong commitment, you need motivation — and a deeper understanding of the weight management program you choose provides some of the tools to keep that motivation strong.

After all, as the cliche goes, in knowledge there is strength. And, to that end, the Polar Fat Free and Fit Forever Program begins your "education" with the basics — in particular, the realities behind the six myths that have long accompanied weight and exercise issues.

MYTH # 1: CUT DOWN YOUR CALORIE INTAKE AND YOU'LL LOSE WEIGHT

It sounds good. Eat less and the weight will drop. And, at a very rudimentary level, it's true. To determine what you need to eat to maintain your present weight, you simply add a zero. For example, if you weighed 150 pounds, your daily caloric intake would be 1,500. To lose weight, you ought to consume less calories than those you need to maintain the status quo. To lose one pound a week, you need to burn 3,500 calories, or 500 calories per day. If you weighed 150 pounds, as in the above example, you'd have to reduce your food intake by 500 calories to lose a pound a week— which would put you on a 1,000 calorie a day diet.

But here's where the problems come in. A 1,000 calorie diet is extremely restrictive; it would be difficult to maintain the discipline you'd need without feeling deprived. Eventually, your motivation would falter and you would get off track.

There are physical ramifications at work here as well. Your body needs a specific number of calories to perform its metabolic functions. When your diet is lower than 1,200 calories per day, your body isn't getting what it needs. Fat cells simply do not supply the amount of glucose, or blood sugar "food" your body needs to

Obesity and Children

More and more, obesity in children is becoming a national problem. Several major studies have found that children's body fat has significantly increased over the past twenty years. There can, of course, be a hereditary link. But there can also be a conditioned link, a habit that begins in childhood — and continues throughout one's adult life. Inactivity. High-fat dining. Sugar snacking. Lack of exercise. All these poor habits are usually taught in childhood.

But, in the same way that you can change a lifetime of bad habits, so can your children. If they follow your new active, healthy example, they too can be assured of a healthier and happier adulthood.

Beth Kirkpatrick, the leading fitness educator for children in the United States, has tested thousands of children with Polar Heart Rate Monitors. She has found that when children exercise with the Polar Heart Rate Monitor, they:

• **Become more fit**
• **Eat healthier**
• **And are motivated to take better care of themselves**

survive on a daily basis. It will soon turn to your lean muscle tissue to get the rest of its glucose requirement. And losing lean muscle tissue will eventually translate into low energy, weakness, loss of muscle tone, and depression.

Yes, you'll show an initial weight loss on a very restrictive diet, but it will be a combination of fat cells and this important lean muscle tissue.

As all this shows, reducing calories alone is not going to do it. But neither is exercise; it's impractical if you live any kind of normal life. You'd have to do an incredible amount of aerobic exercise every day in order to burn 3,500 per week.

There is a better way. And that's a combination of diet and exercise — which is a main component of the Polar Fat Free and Fit Forever Program. In my laboratory, we conducted a landmark diet and exercise study a few years back. We divided 80 people into four groups: a control group who changed nothing during the course of the six-month study, a low-fat diet alone group, an exercise alone group, and a group that combined both diet and exercise. The group that combined diet and exercise had the best results. They:

- Lost an average of 12 pounds — with over 90 percent of it coming from body fat.
- Dropped their blood pressure to within normal ranges.
- Improved their level of fitness, measured by the fact that they consumed more oxygen per minute by the end of the study.
- Experienced a cholesterol drop in their blood.

We followed this study up with yet another. This time, we added strength training. We found that the group that combined a low-fat diet with both aerobic exercise and strength training actually **increased** the lean muscle tissue in their bodies! This translated into more efficient energy production and a higher metabolism — which, in turn, made losing weight and keeping it off a much easier task.

In short, losing weight is more than simply cutting down your calories. It means adding exercise to your life — and the Polar Fat Free and Fit Forever Program will show you how to do this for maximum results.

MYTH # 2: IT DOESN'T MATTER WHAT YOU EAT AS LONG AS IT'S LOW-CALORIE

The amount of food you consume determines the caloric content — not the food itself. After all, no one gains weight from eating one chocolate chip cookie. But different foods do have different calories — and fat has the highest caloric content of all. Gram for gram, fat has more than twice the calories of proteins or carbohydrates. Indeed, it's not the baked potato or the pasta that will add those body fat–increasing calories. It's the butter or sauce that usually accompanies them that can sabotage your weight loss goals.

Obesity is only one result of eating too much fat. Fat, especially saturated fat, has been linked to high blood-cholesterol levels — which, in turn, is a known risk factor in heart disease.

Most of us know that cholesterol can be hazardous to our

health. And yet, the average American consumes between 38% and 40% of his daily calories as fat — and much of that a close encounter of the saturated kind. It makes sense that a recent Surgeon General's Nutrition and Health report claimed that saturated fat is the number one health hazard in the American diet.

We don't recommend eliminating fat from your diet. Some fat is necessary for life — and it cannot be manufactured by our body. Fat aids in the absorption and digestion of certain vitamins; it is a component of our cell tissue; it is a shock absorber, cushioning our bones and vital organs; it insulates us from the cold. Indeed, even the American Heart Association doesn't rule out fat entirely. But it does recommend restricting fat to no more than 30% of your daily calories. Further, it recommends that you use polyunsaturated and monosaturated fats whenever possible — both of which tend to lower cholesterol levels.

The Polar Fat Free and Fit Forever Program keeps within these American Heart Association guidelines. It is a program literally for life — as you will see.

MYTH # 3: THE HARDER YOU EXERCISE, THE BETTER IT IS

This myth is synonymous with the masochist's credo, "No pain, no gain." Granted, you sometimes have to work hard to get what you want, but staying focused has little to do with strenuous labor or pain. In fact, the groundbreaking longitudinal Framingham, Massachussetts study which followed more than 5,000 residents for 25 years found that the best results from exercise occurred within people who just started moving. In other words, simply getting off the couch and going for a stroll a few times a week provides excellent results for beginners.

A good workout requires three elements — none of which have anything to do with pain:

■ **Endurance.** The length of time you can exercise at one clip is a crucial factor. The longer the time, the better. Performing less strenuous exercise, such as walking, means you can keep at it much longer than if you jumped up off the couch and tried to run a mile. We guarantee you wouldn't get far — and you certainly wouldn't try it again soon.

■ **Intensity.** It's true that a hard workout will get results, but only if you are in shape — and only if you are not pushing yourself. Running, working out on an exercise machine or stationary cycle — even walking — can be potentially dangerous if you are exercising past your fitness level or overexerting yourself.

■ **Frequency.** One burst of energy isn't going to do it. For long-term fitness, you need to exercise at least three times a week at your fitness level. And the only way you'll keep with it is if you are motivated — which can only be sustained if you are not overexerting yourself and you are not experiencing pain.

In short, the best exercises are those that enable you ...

1. to work out several times a week for an extended period of time...
2. to work at a level effective for you to lose weight and maintain cardiovascular health.

"YO-YO" Dieting

A slow metabolism spells survival in primitive cultures — where a restrictive diet isn't by choice. To ward off starvation, the body slows down the rate at which it burns whatever calories are consumed. This slower metabolism helps conserve a dwindling energy reserve from lack of food. In today's civilized world, however, our bodies can't tell the difference between starvation and restrictive dieting. The more you stay on your diet, the more your body will slow down your metabolism — and the harder it will be to lose weight.

The harder the diet becomes, the harder it is to stay with it. Add food behavior that has not changed and a poor body image to the equation, and it's only a matter of time before the weight is all gained back — with the slower metabolism in place to boot.

The solution for a great many dieters? Another "crash" diet — that will ultimately fail. It's no accident that "yo-yo" dieting has become a way of life for many — or that 95 percent of the people who lose weight gain it back within two years.

And the key to this type of exercise is the target heart rate zone — or, as we call it, the weight management zone.

The target heart rate zone, or weight management zone, is the foundation behind the Polar Fat Free and Fit Forever Program. Research has found that exercising at an intensity that puts you in this zone — not more and not less — is the most effective place for you to burn calories, help your heart, and maintain long-term health **without** risk of injury. Exercising in your target heart rate zone is recommended by the American Heart Association, the American

College of Sports Medicine, and by leading fitness testing centers, universities, cardiologists, cardiac rehabilitation centers, physiologists and weight loss experts across the country. You can reach your weight management zone by doing any exercise — whether it be walking or running, using a stationary cycle or a stair-stepper, aerobic class or swimming, bicycling or strength training. It's not the exercise: it's the target heart rate zone that counts. We'll "zone" in on this in much more detail in the next few chapters. We'll also help you find your ideal weight management zone — and show you where the Polar Heart Rate Monitor fits in to ensure you are working out for maximum pain-free results.

MYTH # 4: OBESITY IS A MINOR HEALTH RISK FACTOR

Do you remember the expression, "Fat people are happy"? Anyone who is overweight knows this is a lie. On a par with this cliche is obesity's role in ill health. Only ten years ago, being overweight was either discounted or considered a minor health risk. Today, we know better. Obesity is not only an underlying factor in conditions — such as hypertension, diabetes, inactivity, and high cholesterol — that lead to heart disease, it can, like these conditions, lead directly to heart disease itself. Further, the 1989 Surgeon General report stated that seven out of the ten leading causes of death in the United States were related to alcohol abuse or poor nutrition — with obesity a major factor in poor nutrition. In other words, cut out the fat and the health risk decreases. Here is some evidence:

■ The Coronary Heart Disease (CHD) Link

In 1992, the researchers in a 15 year study of 117,000 nurses, called the National Nurses Cooperative Trial, found that there was a significant relationship between obesity and CHD. In fact, the more overweight a person was, the stronger the association. Even more sobering was the evidence that being a mere 15 pounds overweight throughout one's lifetime substantially increased a woman's risk of heart disease.

All Fats Are Not Created Equal

SATURATED FAT	MONOUNSATURATED	POLYUNSATURATED
Butter	Olive Oil	Safflower oil
Dairy fat	Peanut Oil	Sunflower oil
Beef fat	Canola oil	Corn oil
Lard		Soybean oil
Chicken fat		Cottonseed oil
Vegetable shortening		Margarine (made
Hydrogenated vegetable oil		with liquid oil)
Palm oil		
Palm kernel oil		
Coconut oil		
Cocoa butter (found in chocolate)		

NOTE: Chart taken from *The Rockport Walking Program* by Dr. James M. Rippe, Ann Ward, Ph.D., with Karla Dougherty, New York: Fireside Press, 1989, page 10

■ The Hypertension Link

The connection between obesity and high blood pressure is well-established. A person can lower his blood pressure by one millimeter of mercury for every two pounds he loses — and that weight loss might be all he needs to keep his blood pressure in check. In fact, the first thing I do when I see a hypertensive patient who is overweight is insist he lose weight.

And, in following a diet program to lose weight, my patients also initiate other healthful actions: they lower their salt intake and stop eating as much high-fat food. The Polar Fat Free and Fit Forever Program already factors in these healthier eating habits. And, with its emphasis on activity in a specific weight management zone, it also promotes another factor in lower blood pressure: aerobic exercise.

■ The Elevated Cholesterol Link

Cholesterol is a waxy substance manufactured by your body that is vital for many of its functions. It is a natural substance found in all animal products, from steak and eggs to margarine, and it is also a by-product of consuming saturated fat. The more animal-originated foods and saturated fats we eat, the more that cholesterol can build up and block up arteries — leading to CHD.

Lipoproteins, made of protein and fat in the liver, carry cholesterol through our bodies. The majority of lipoproteins are LDL, or low-density lipoprotein cholesterol. Unfortunately, LDL can build up to dangerous levels, either through genetics or bad eating habits. Once the body "takes" what it needs, removing and

Finding the Hidden Fat
In Your Supermarket

Beware the words "Lite" or "Low-Calorie." The government is in the process of making companies provide clearer food labels on their packages, but in the meantime, here are some suggestions to help you steer clear of unwanted fat:

1. Always check your labels. Notice exactly what the calorie count is — and the grams of fat per serving. Here's a simple equation to figure out how the percentage of fat in each serving, using a slice (one serving) of smoked cooked ham, which has 25 calories and 1 gram of fat, as an example:

   a. Multiply the grams of fat by 9.
      (1 gram of fat X 9 = 9)

   b. Divide your result by the number of calories per serving. (9 divided by 25 calories = .36)

   c. Multiply this result by 100. (.36 X 100 = 36%)

      Try to choose food items that get less than half their calories from fat. In the above example, the smoked cooked ham is a good choice: only 36%, or less than half, of its calories come from fat per serving.

2. Beware the word hydrogenation — which turns unsaturated liquid oils into saturated fat.

3. Liquid oil should be the first ingredient on a margarine's label. And it should contain twice the amount of polyunsaturated fat than saturated fat.

4. Don't be fooled by "no cholesterol." Legally, a food product can proclaim this if it has no animal product. But, remember, foods with no cholesterol can still have a lot of saturated fat. Vegetable shortening, coconut oil, all these can hold "hidden" fat.

absorbing the LDL from the artery passageways, the remaining LDL continues to "float" in the bloodstream, eventually depositing its load of cholesterol and fat on the artery walls and clogging them. This is why LDL is considered "bad" cholesterol.

HDL, or high-density lipoprotein cholesterol, is "good" cholesterol. Like a high-tech vacuum cleaner, HDL removes the cholesterol residue left by LDL; it carries it back to the liver.

One excellent way to reduce cholesterol build-up is to lose weight — which decreases both the amount of fat in your body, particularly the "bad" LDL-linked saturated fat, and the amount of cholesterol in your blood. The combination of aerobic exercise, which promotes the manufacture of good HDL-cholesterol, and a sound weight loss program, such as the Polar Fat Free and Fit Forever Program, can effectively reduce this risk.

■ The Quality of Life Link

The risk of physical disease is not the only danger involved in obesity. Obesity can also create:

Anxiety and depression. If you eat when you are anxious or depressed, you are not alone. It is a way of coping with life's stresses, one that you most likely have used for a long, long time. The only problem is that the food/anxiety connection feeds upon itself. The more you eat, the worse you feel — especially if the food you are reaching for is filled with sugar and fat.

The Physician and Sports Medicine study of 1,751 primary-care doctors found that 80 percent of them prescribed exercise for depression and 60 percent prescribed it for anxiety. Further, a walking study we did at the Exercise Physiology Lab found that each person significantly reduced her anxiety and tension and elevated her overall mood for at least two hours after walking — regardless of fitness level or speed!

Poor appearance, self-esteem, and overall emotional state. The heavier you are, the less inclined you are to get up and get moving. Maybe you don't want to go out and face the world. Maybe you simply don't have the energy. Whatever it is, obesity is an all-pervasive factor in your poor emotional state. Get rid of the fat, begin to eat healthfully, start walking — and watch both your appearance and your mood improve.

A healthy lifestyle really does keep people mentally and physically young. With the heart rate monitor as a built-in motivational tool, the Polar Fat Free and Fit Forever Program is designed to help everyone get up off the sofa and change their life — for good.

The Setpoint Theory

Setpoint is directly related to the slower metabolism that comes from too restricted a diet. It is an internal thermostat within the brain that decides how many fat cells a person should have; each person has their own setpoint and it is as individual as the thermostat you set in your own house. If you are overweight, this setpoint has, most likely, been set at your current weight — especially if you've been on a lose weight/gain it back "yo-yo" treadmill. Try to lose any weight — and this setpoint gets the body to fight you every step of the way until it's all been gained back. In fact, the only way to keep weight off is to reset your setpoint control to a lower fat cell requirement — through exercise.

MYTH # 5: A HEALTHY, STRONG HEART IS INHERITED — AND A MATTER OF GENES

Your physical make-up, your ability to handle stress, your predisposition for certain diseases — all these are affected by the genes that have been passed on to you.

Your genes can also transfer specific coronary diseases, certain inherited valve problems and cardiac arhythmias that are serious and cannot be changed. But, these conditions aside, heredity does not create a pre-ordained fate when it comes to heart disease. Indeed, heredity is only one factor.

Coronary heart disease is also a result of bad habits **that can change.** The proof comes from the longitudinal Framingham, Massachussetts study. By following the 5,000 Framingham residents for more than 25 years, researchers have been able to determine the risk factors involved in CHD — most of which are based on bad habits. These risk factors are:

1. High blood pressure, or hypertension

2. Elevated cholesterol

3. Cigarette smoking

4. Sedentary lifestyle

5. Stress

6. Obesity

7. Diabetes

8. Family history of coronary artery disease

As you can see, only one of these factors is related to inherited genes.

There are reasons why a healthy heart is influenced by habits we can change. Despite the soul-searching words and deeply-felt emotion that "heart" conveys to poets and philosophers, it is, in reality, a "hard body" muscle — a pump that looks like a tight fist. This fist, however, packs a mighty wallop, continuously surging twelve pints of blood through our system. In an average person, the strength of this "squirting blood" is comparable to turning on the water faucet full blast. This "jet" of blood squirting through your system can be felt as a pulse. Each beat of your pulse pushes out approximately one cup of blood into your system.

The pumping action is a result of contractions or heart beats. When the heart is not contracting, it is at rest. Blood can flow into its various chambers and fill up. When the heart contracts, this blood is "pushed" and pumped out into the bloodstream. This pumping action is involuntary; the contractions are regulated by a natural pacemaker located in the heart. But the rate at which the contractions occur varies from person to person. The more fit an individual, the lower the resting heart rate — which puts less strain on the heart. Conversely, the less fit you are, the higher the resting heart rate — and the more strain that is put on the heart. (We'll be going over this in more detail in the next chapter.)

Exercise can help make you fit — and make your heart strong. The Polar Fat Free and Fit Forever Program will help you find the maximum fitness level you can use to lose weight without straining your heart. It will help you find your individual weight management zone where you will get the best results — without hurting yourself. And the Polar Heart Rate Monitor will also help you actually control your heart beats — in an instant form of biofeedback.

Oxygen and You

Your body needs oxygen to live and, the more fit you are, the better and more efficient it is to transport this "food" to each and every cell. Our maximal aerobic capacity is called VO2MAX, which stands for Maximum Oxygen Consumption. Exercising at 60 to 70 percent of your own individual VO2MAX will:

1. Improve your heart's ability to pump oxygenated blood throughout your system.

2. Help your muscles better extract oxygen from this oxygen-rich blood traveling through your system.

Both these factors translate into a higher aerobic capacity and more energy to perform your daily chores.

Seventy to 80 percent of your VO2MAX is inherited but you can improve what you've got with exercise — especially the kind of effective exercise you'll get by using your Polar Heart Rate Monitor.

MYTH # 6: BY THE TIME YOU HIT MIDDLE AGE, IT'S TOO LATE TO CHANGE YOUR LIFESTYLE

If you come away learning one thing within the pages of this book, we hope it will be the knowledge that you can make changes in your life. You can change the way you look and feel at any age. A 50-year-old woman wanted to participate in our studies at the Exercise Physiology Lab because she felt — and looked — older than she wanted to. Within a few months of eating a low-fat diet and exercising within her weight management zone three to five days a week, her entire outlook completely changed. Not only was there a glow to her cheeks and a vibrancy to her step, but she felt healthier. She felt positive about her life — despite the same stresses that were there three months before she started her new regime.

This woman is only one of many who have seen that age is a state of mind — that can be changed. A study conducted a few years back researched both active and inactive women between two age groups: 70 to 79 and 19 to 20. In terms of reaction time, balance, and strength, the active older women between the ages of 70 and 79 most resembled the young, active 19–20 year olds — rather than the inactive women their own age!

In short, age is more a function of inactivity than the actual aging process. We can't promise that the Polar Fat Free and Fit

Forever Program will be a fountain of youth, but we do guarantee that, if you read this book and follow our guidelines, you will feel healthier and more in control of yourself than you have in years.

To that end, let us now leave these fitness and nutrition myths and, armed with your newfound knowledge, go on to the actual Polar Fat Free and Fit Forever Program — and the first step towards beginning your own individual Polar Program: understanding the principles that make up the Polar Fat Free and Fit Forever Program. **Onward. . . .**

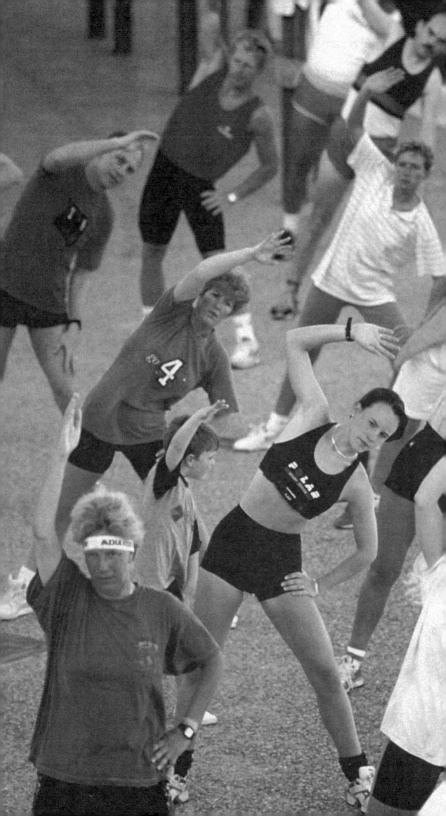

Losing Weight
With The
Polar
Fat Free
and
Fit Forever
Program

*"I've lost twelve pounds already in three months —
and it was so easy, I don't even feel like I was trying!"*

—A 45-year-old housewife on the Polar Program for the first time

■ Jeanne never thought she could lose the weight she gained after giving birth to her two children. She'd tried everything, from group meetings to packaged foods, from liquid shakes to one-on-one counseling. Nothing ever did the trick — until her husband bought her a Polar Heart Rate Monitor for her birthday. Suddenly, the exercise — not the restricted diet — came first. Jeanne began to walk. And walk. Three times a week. No one had to drag her; she wanted to do her exercise. Strapping on her heart rate monitor and checking her progress turned out to be fun. And, suddenly, it also became easier and easier to eat low-fat foods. Suddenly, exercise became a part of her life. So did the Polar Fat Free and Fit Forever Program.

■ Sam didn't remember when his life wasn't stressful. He enjoyed his work, but he worked hard. Too hard to fit in more than a sporadic workout at his health club here and there. Things changed when his physician told him his blood pressure was up and his cholesterol was elevated. Sam decided it was time for a major change in his life. He bought a Polar Heart Rate Monitor and read about its simple exercise and diet combination for long-term health. He began the program with a vengeance. Every time he used the Lifecycle, on would go the Polar. Every time he worked out with weights, on would go the Polar. He stopped eating saturated fat. And, soon, he began to feel better than he had in years. The next doctor visit? His blood pressure and cholesterol levels were down — all without medication.

■ Margaret had reached a slump in her fitness plan. She felt she was in reasonably good shape since she'd already lost thirty pounds and regularly walked three times a week. But she still had those last ten pounds to lose. And she wanted to maintain her fitness level. Lately, she'd begun to slip. A cookie here. A fatty salad dressing there. And the weekly walking was moving down to only two times. She needed something — and that something was the Polar Fat Free and Fit Forever Program. A friend bought her a heart rate monitor for Christmas. She found it easy to use — and she realized that she'd spent the last few months in a lower heart rate zone than her new fitness level prescribed. No wonder she wasn't losing more weight. No wonder she wasn't feeling challenged. Soon, Margaret had pushed herself into her new, more appropriate walking zone. She combined her new exercise regime with the Polar nutrition plan — and those tough last ten pounds seemed to melt away.

• • • • • • • • •

These people are like many others who have tried the Polar Fat Free and Fit Forever Program — and found it easy to follow, easy to use and easy to be successful. We've already expelled those common fat and exercise myths. Now it's time to begin the Polar Way. To that end, here are the four sound principles behind the program, principles that, once they are in your grasp, will keep your motivation strong and your success rate high.

POLAR PRINCIPLE # 1:
THE POLAR EFFECTIVE ENERGY EQUATION

I t's basic math, as easy as 1 + 1 = 2. In order for a weight management program to be effective, you must burn more calories than you eat. Simple. But as we have seen in Chapter One, decreasing your food intake isn't enough. True, you take in less calories, but you also end up burning more than fat. You end up losing vital muscle tone.

Nor is exercise alone a good solution. You'd have to exercise an extraordinary amount each week in order to offset the amount of food you've always eaten.

The best answer to the energy equation is and always will be a combination of diet and exercise. As we have seen in Chapter One, studies performed at our Exercise Physiology Lab and at other research centers show that this combination is the most efficient, effective, and conclusive way to lose weight.

TAKE IT TO THE VO2MAX

Exercise and diet work together in the energy equation, true, but people are not numbers. No two people will have the same requirements — whether it be the amount of food they eat, the energy they need to expend, or the type of exercise they want to do. Each person is an individual—with his or her own individual equation for efficient weight loss and health.

The key to that individuality comes from fitness — which is measured by VO2MAX. As we have seen in the previous chapter VO2MAX, or Maximum Oxygen Consumption, is the maximum amount of oxygen you consume per minute. Here's how it works: When you exercise, your muscles "request" energy. Your brain, hearing their call, stimulates the heart to deliver oxygen to these demanding muscles — via the red blood cells. Once distributed to your muscles, this oxygen combines with glucose, glycogen, and free fatty acids; it is broken down by enzymes, consumed, and, ultimately, used in the production of more energy.

When you exercise at 60 percent to 80 percent of your VO2MAX, you are actually over-stressing your system — which is good. It means that you are increasing your heart's ability to pump oxygen-rich blood throughout your body; it means you are helping your muscles become more efficient at extracting the oxygen as the blood flows along. The result? Physical activities, such as shoveling the snow, climbing the stairs, or running for a bus, will no longer wear you out.

The better your shape, the higher your VO2MAX. An average 20-year-old woman's VO2MAX will be between 35 and 40 milliliters for every kilogram of her body weight per minute — if she's exercising at her maximum capacity. But a top marathon runner will have a VO2MAX around 70 milliliters for that same kilogram of body weight per minute.

The Diet and Exercise Combination: A Good Fit

- **The Polar study we conducted at the Exercise Physiology Lab showed our subjects lost an average of eight pounds of fat, or a 10 percent decrease in body fat — and actually gained calorie-burning lean muscle tissue.**

- **A study performed as early as 1979 found that a diet alone group lost seven pounds, an exercise alone group lost six pounds — but a group that combined both diet and exercise lost 13 pounds!**

- **Two month and six month follow-ups in that same early study found that the exercise and diet group was the only one to continue to lose weight.**

- **The walking study we performed at the Exercise Physiology Lab in 1989 confirmed these same facts: the group that combined both walking and a low-fat diet lost more weight and body fat than the diet alone and exercise alone groups — with no loss of lean muscle tissue.**

Although the bulk of your VO2MAX capability is inherited, you can improve what you've got — with exercise. At our Exercise Physiology Laboratory, we've proven that a simple aerobic activity such as walking will increase VO2MAX in people of all ages — and at all levels of fitness.

Although you need to know your VO2MAX to begin an exercise program at an appropriate level, we've done the work for you. In the next chapter, you'll find a Polar Aerobic Fitness Test which will estimate your initial VO2MAX. This means that you will be able to begin the exercise of your choice on the Polar Program at the right level, not too high so you'll get injured or lose motivation — nor too low so you won't get the important health and weight loss benefits.

The BMR Connection

Here's another reason for a moderate exercise and diet regime like the Polar Fat Free and Fit Forever Program. Basal metabolic rate (BMR) is a term used by scientists and exercise physiologists to denote the amount of energy your body burns when it is at rest. When you eat less food, your BMR drops. Indeed, very restrictive diets can drop your BMR by as much as 45 percent. This means that you're simply not going to burn as many calories when you are at rest. Hence, the diet plateaus, discouragement, and, ultimately, weight gains found on very restrictive diets.

TARGET HEART-RATE ZONE (BEATS/MIN)

AGE (YRS)	TARGET ZONE (BEATS/MIN)				AVERAGE MAX HR (100%)
	50%	60%	70%	80%	
20	100	120	140	170	200
25	98	117	137	166	195
30	95	114	133	162	190
35	93	111	130	157	185
40	90	108	126	153	180
45	88	105	123	149	175
50	85	102	119	145	170
55	83	99	116	140	165
60	80	96	112	136	160
65	78	93	109	132	155
70	75	90	105	128	150

AEROBIC EXERCISE AND RESISTANCE TRAINING

But there's still more to this energy equation than efficiently burning calories at your individual fitness level. There's the actual exercise you do as well. Aerobic exercise literally means "in the presence of air," as your large muscle groups continuously and rhythmically use oxygen for at least twenty minutes at a clip. Your Polar Heart Rate Monitor helps you maintain your appropriate aerobic intensity which, in turn, translates into:

- A loss of body fat while preserving lean muscle tissue
- Efficient calorie burning
- Decreased appetite
- Improved mood and decreased anxiety — which means you'll stay with your program, feeling motivated, proud, and in control.

Although it doesn't burn calories as efficiently as the energy equation specifies, resistance strength training is just as important.

(NOTE: Chart taken from *The Rockport Walking Program* by Dr. James M. Rippe, Ann Ward, Ph.D., with Karla Dougherty, New York: Fireside Press, 1989, page 51)

Resistance strength training is the only way I know to actually increase your lean muscle tissue. Further, you can increase the size of your calorie-burning engine — which will translate into better weight management. And the feeling of strength, of firm, toned muscles will make you want to get out there and walk... run...swim...live!

Fat Burning Zone: Fact or Fiction?

There is no magic zone for burning fat. Many people have misconstrued the fact that at lower levels of exercise, you burn a higher proportion of fat. They've labeled this lower level a "fat burning zone" and placed it right below the aerobic training zone. Yes, it's true that lower levels will burn calories, but it's not because of a special exercise zone. The reason a lower level of exercise works is because beginners keep coming back. It is the most comfortable zone for beginners, a level they can accomplish, where they can get the exercise they need at an intensity that will not hurt — and that makes them feel good. The result? They will come back for more, working out a healthy, fat-burning three to five times a week. Sixty percent to 70 percent is a good place to start for this purpose. We call it the *Weight Management Zone* — a target heart rate area where you can exercise for long periods of time, a place where you can burn the maximum number of fat-producing calories with the greatest degree of comfort.

THE METABOLIC FACTOR

Muscle is the most metabolically active tissue in your body. It can also be said to be metabolically sensitive. We've already seen how a poor diet and exercise regime will result in a slower metabolism — that can be set for life. Age, too, can lower your metabolism. As you get older, your muscles gradually shrink, at about a half a pound a year after thirty. This small half-pound loss can result in a slowdown of your resting metabolism of approximately .5 percent a year. This means that although you might be eating the same amount of food, you're burning it more slowly — and accumulating fat.

Exercise, on the other hand, has been found to raise metabolic rates for up to four hours after an aerobic exercise session is over — which means more energy and more burned up calories.

TARGETING YOUR WEIGHT MANAGEMENT ZONE

Weight loss success and long-term health comes down to two short words: heart rate. It's everything we've been working up to in our discussion so far and it's at the crux of the Polar Fat Free and Fit Forever Program. As we have seen in Chapter One, your heart beat is regulated by your natural pacemaker; your beats per minute (bpm) are automatic. The rate varies from person to person; this variation is a result of a person's fitness level, one's cardiovascular chemistry — even an anxious moment can make one's heart beat faster.

To recap: Your heart rate is the signal that blood is being pumped through your system. The more fit you are, the stronger your beating heart pumps oxygen-rich blood through your body and the more efficient your muscles are in absorbing that oxygen from the blood. The result is a higher metabolism, greater calories burned, and more energy, vibrancy, and health.

Great. We know a good working heart rate is important for cardiovascular health and weight loss. But where do you start? How do you know what heart rate is best for maximum results?

There is no one number that you should aim for. Rather, there are four target heart rate exercise zones that will improve your health, weight management, fitness, and even peak performance. And one of them is right for you.

Each target heart rate exercise zone is based on a percentage of your Maximum Heart Rate (MHR), which means exactly as it sounds: the maximum number of times your heart beats, or contracts, in one minute. Your MHR is determined by subtracting your age from 220. (For example, if you were 40 years old, your MHR would be 220 − 40 = 180 beats per minute.) Refer to the table opposite to determine the various target heart rate zones. The target heart rate zone you ultimately choose is dependent upon your level of fitness:

■ 50 percent to 60 percent of your MHR is considered the **Moderate Activity Zone.** This is a good place for beginners and people who have not exercised in a long time to start.

■ We call 60 to 70 percent of your MHR the **Weight Management Zone.** You will most likely know it well by the time

TARGET HEART RATE EXERCISE ZONES

**Exercise in your proper target heart rate zone for improved
health, weight management, fitness and peak performance.**

% Of Maximum Heart Rate	Target Heart Rate Zone
50 – 60%	Moderate Activity*
60 – 70%	Weight Management
70 – 80%	Aerobic Training
80 – 100%	Competitive Training

*** The American College of Sports Medicine and The Centers for Disease
Control and Prevention recommend 30 minutes or more of moderate-
intensity physical activity at least three times a week to improve
overall health.**

**Please note: Be sure to do warm-up exercise at a target heart rate zone
that is lower than the zones in the table above. Exercise for five to ten
minutes in this lower zone prior to exercising in the target heart rate
zone you select. Also, remember to cool down for five to ten minutes
after exercising. Use a lower target heart rate zone than the zone you
selected for your exercise.**

you're into your first month on the Polar Program. This is the target
heart rate zone that, for most of you, will be the optimum place to
start to burn fat and get your heart rate up to a level which will result
in a better level of fitness with minimal aerobic exercise.

■ 70 to 80 percent of your MHR is the **Aerobic Training Zone.**
After you've been on the Polar Program for several weeks, you
might be ready to move up to this zone. It's a place for the average
fit person who works out on a regular basis.

■ 80 to 100 percent of your MHR is a rare place, reserved for
professional athletes and those gifted with an innate high VO2MAX.
It is called the **Competitive Training Zone** and, the more Polar

becomes a part of your life, the more you can aspire to reach at least the low end of this "rainbow."

POLAR PRINCIPLE # 2:
POLAR PRECISION TRAINING

For the best results in your Polar Program — and in any program, for that matter — accuracy is crucial. From exercising in your weight management zone to following the correct Polar calorie plan, you need to be accurate. If you don't know whether you are in your target heart rate zone or maintaining it during your session, you might not be burning enough calories to lose weight — or you might be overexerting yourself and vulnerable to injury.

Accuracy is also part of the training process. In order to achieve your personal best, to go beyond the starter zones, you need to know exactly how you are doing. You have to have an accurate heart rate reading in order to know when you are ready to go further. You have to know that the ease with which you might be walking, the lack of challenge in your step, the low level exertion you feel on the stationary cycle, is, in reality, the need to go to a higher heart rate zone — and not an inaccurate reading of your current one.

Before Polar invented the Polar Heart Rate Monitor, there were only two ways to determine whether or not you were in your target heart rate zone.

You could stop in your tracks, check your watch, and take your pulse. Unfortunately, the reading might not be accurate.

Once you stop what you are doing, your pulse immediately drops. And relying on a watch and some quick mathematics is not ideal in terms of accuracy. Worse, some people have difficulty finding their pulse.

The second method for target heart rate zones relies on your own "take", based on levels of exertion. If you are tired, out of breath, or in pain, you would pull back. If, on the other hand, you felt like you were out on a stroll, you'd push yourself further. This is fine for someone who's been working out for a while — and who doesn't need to lose weight. However, beginners and those in training alike need accuracy for best results. They need to know that they are doing the best they can do.

Today there is a better way.

TARGETING MADE EASIER: THE POLAR HEART RATE MONITOR

The Polar Heart Rate Monitor is your key to success. It's the reason why this program is different from any other. It's the reason why you will have success on the Polar Program — even if you've tried other diet and exercise programs before.

In the next chapter, you'll take an easy Polar Fitness Test in the exercise of your choice and, armed with your results, you'll learn what target heart rate zone to aim for and maintain. The Polar Heart Rate Monitor will help you accurately and efficiently stay within that zone. Because it is a visible aid, a fast, easy way to see if you are in your target heart rate zone, you also get immediate feedback — which will go far in keeping your motivation strong.

As you already know, I feel very strongly about Polar Heart Rate Monitors. We've been using them for years at the Exercise Physiology and Nutrition Lab. I like to think of them as a "window to your heart" because, in a very real sense, you are visualizing in a very direct way what is going on with your heart during exercise. And, because the heart rate monitor is keyed to your own individual rate, it will display the subtle changes that go on from day to day in your exercise regime, helping you chart an accurate individualized course. Whether you are tired or energized, cold or hot, soaking wet or parched — these and any other variables will show up in the way you perform and, ultimately, on your heart rate monitor.

Think of your Polar Heart Rate Monitor as your personal trainer, something that provides that extra push, that makes the mind/body link real. As you exercise, you begin to feel better — both mentally and physically. As you're walking or swimming or cycling, you look down. And there, on your wrist, is the feedback — and reinforcement — you need to keep going. You're feeling good and you know why: you're in your target heart rate zone.

You're growing strong.

But don't just take my word for it. Here are some study results that prove the continuous and accurate feedback you get from your heart rate monitor works:

■ A study conducted at Columbia University found that those subjects who did not have feedback while exercising on a stationary bicycle stayed in their target heart rate zone only 51.1 percent of the time. Those who did have heart rate feedback stayed within their zone **87.2 percent.**

■ When we compared heart rates derived from taking a pulse to a heart rate monitor at the Exercise Physiology Lab, we found that 60 percent of aerobic instructors were unable to get an accurate reading from their pulse during warm-up, aerobics, or cool-down.

WHY POLAR?

The Polar Fat Free and Fit Forever Program uses the heart rate monitor for its exercise component because:

1. It provides comfort. By remaining in your appropriate target heart rate zone, you'll avoid injury — and want to stay with your exercise regime.

2. It offers safety. By accurately knowing that you are in your target heart rate zone, you will maximize the safety feature of the Polar Program.

3. It is precise. Direct measurement of your heart rate during exercise is simply the most accurate way to insure you achieve your goals.

4. It keeps you motivated. Comfort, safety, and precision add up to one very important long-term goal for success: motivation. If you are comfortable and seeing real progress being made, you will enjoy what you are doing. Enjoy what you are doing and you'll be motivated. It's that simple.

POLAR PRINCIPLE # 3:
A NUTRITIONALLY-SOUND, EASY-TO-FOLLOW DIET EXCHANGE

xercising with your heart rate monitor is only one component of the Polar Fat Free and Fit Forever Program. In order to lose weight and live healthfully, you must also eat healthfully. When you hear the word "diet," it might conjure up thoughts of deprivation and plates full of carrots morning, noon, and night. Not so with the Polar Program. We don't believe you must eat less food — just fewer calories and **better** food for your body.

The Polar Fat Free and Fit Forever Program is based on the American Heart Association and the American Dietetic Association's guidelines. We recommend that only 23 percent to 30 percent of your daily intake be in fats — with an avoidance, as much as possible, of saturated fats. We also recommend foods rich in fiber, including fresh fruits and vegetables, and complex carbohydrates.

The daily caloric requirements you need is based on the amount of exercise you do. The Polar Fat Free and Fit Forever Program offers three meal plans, either 1,200 calories a day, 1,500 calories a day, or 1,800 calories a day. Based on your current weight and exercise regime, you'll choose one of these groups for a healthy, gradual weight loss of approximately one to two pounds a week — and we'll show you exactly how this works in Chapter Five.

We've done the work for you in the Polar Nutrition Program. Instead of spending your time figuring out how many calories are in the sandwich you are about to eat, we've divided foods into six categories. Within each category are lists of food that can be exchanged from one to the other. For example, in the starch/bread category, a 1 oz. four-grain roll can be substituted for a 1/2 cup of rigatoni. Each of these food servings are called an "exchange" and you have a specific amount of exchanges from each category that you must eat each day. (You will find the complete lists of food exchanges within each category at the back of this book.) The six food categories are:

- Starch/Bread
- Protein/Meat
- Vegetable
- Fruit
- Milk
- Fat

The food exchange system was developed by the American Dietetic Association and the American Diabetes Association. We've used it in all of our major weight management research projects and we know it works.

The Polar Program makes the dieting plan as easy as the exercise plan. With an exchange system, there's no calories to count and you have the added plus of flexibility. If you want an orange instead of an apple, fine. It's one exchange either way. If you are going to a big party one night, no problem. Save most of your daily exchanges for the evening and you can sample the hors d'oeuvres and even have a glass of wine. In short, with this diet plan, there's no deprivation or sacrifice. It's something you can live with for the rest of your life. After all what can be more life-sustaining and positive than incorporating healthy eating into your new-found exercise routine!

PRINCIPLE # 4:
LONG-TERM MOTIVATION

Short-term motivation is easy. Ask anyone who's just started a diet. There's always a determined burst of resolve at the beginning of any new diet and exercise program, a wish to do things just right. But ask that same person a few weeks into the regime and you might hear a different story. Maybe they feel deprived. Maybe they're dragging their heels. Maybe they just sound plain bored. Whatever it is, keeping that motivation strong over the long run is definitely the hard part. Sticking with a plan and maintaining your weight loss can be a challenge without the right tools.

Quite frankly, the only way a plan can work is through a change of lifestyle and a change of behavior. This takes what I call the **3M Pledge for Behavior Change** and it's the basis of this last principle in the Polar Fat Free and Fit Forever Program:

■ **Motivation...** means finding the personal will to change. The Polar Heart Rate Monitor, incorporated into your exercise regime, helps keep your exercise motivation high. Combined with an easy-to-follow, non-deprivation diet plan and my sound philosophy for behavior change, it makes a powerful "charge" for change. I am confident that you're simply going to feel so much better, be so much more in control of your life, and lose weight so painlessly with the Polar Fat Free and Fit Forever Program that your motivation will continue to stay strong until you've reached your long-term health and weight goals — and beyond.

■ **Measurement...** means keeping track of your performance. You need to measure where you stand right now, before you begin the Polar Program, and at ten and twenty week intervals during your "training." The self-tests in the next chapter will measure your initial fitness and weight loss goals; they will help you start off at the level that is best for you. By measuring your food and your exercise routines as you go along, you'll see improvements fast — and you'll know when it's time to reach for the next fitness level or meal plan. Measuring is built into the Polar Way. We provide sample exercise logs and food diaries to help you get off to the right start — to insure long-lasting behavior change motivation and stick-with-it motivation.

■ **Maintenance...** is the key to long-term weight management. The skills you learn and the lifestyle changes you make form the foundation for far-reaching weight control. The fact that you feel happier, more energetic, and proud of yourself on the Polar Program assures that this "M" — and the entire 3M Pledge — takes place.

•   •   •   •   •   •   •   •

Okay. You now have all the groundwork in place to begin the Polar Fat Free and Fit Forever Program. It's time now to actually begin your own individualized regime. And in the next chapter, you'll learn where to start — and how . . . .

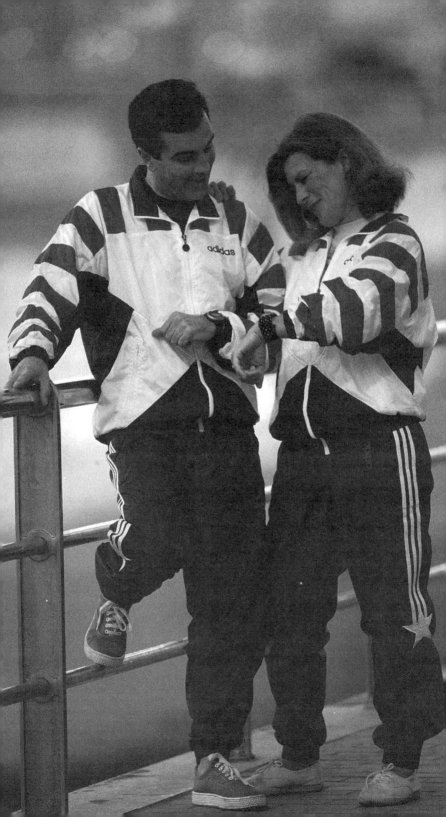

The Polar Program Tests

"For the first time ever I feel in control of my life."

—A 56-year-old woman
who has just started the Polar Fat Free and Fit Forever Program

Testing can be a powerful tool. By testing yourself

before you start the Polar Fat Free and Fit Forever Program, you will

be assured of starting at a level that's right for you. You'll also be

able to formulate your weight and fitness goals.

But there's more. When you take the same tests again a few

weeks from now, you'll receive a strong incentive to go on —

because you will see, in plain black and white, that you've

improved.

So, without further ado, let's go to a battery of self-tests that we've designed to help you assess your body fat, aerobic capacity, and current eating habits. These four tests are simple to do and they can even be enjoyable. All you need is a little time and a pad and pencil to jot down your answers which will be used to set up your personal Polar Program.

THE POLAR BODY FAT MEASUREMENT TEST

The problem of obesity is really a problem of excess body **fat.** If you are overweight, you need to lose your extra **fat** — while preserving your lean muscle tissue. Standard height and weight charts do not distinguish between body fat and lean muscle. The chart might show that 166 pounds is the standard weight for a six-foot tall man, but it doesn't take the weight of his muscles into account. A very muscular man, for example, may weight 190 pounds, but not be overweight because he has a low percentage of body fat. On the other hand, an unathletic man with the same height and weight would be 14 pounds overweight because his extra pounds are almost all in body fat.

Unfortunately, most of us have lived under the shadow of height and weight charts, using the scale as the Great Indicator of how much we've gained or lost. We've been unable to separate body fat from muscle, only seeing numbers that, in reality, mean little. There is a better way, one that measures body fat only.

In the laboratory setting, we have precise tools to distinguish between lean muscle tissue and body fat. Underwater weighing is used most often for research purposes; it takes advantage of the

The Scales of Dieting

Exercise, water retention, stress, body chemistry — all these can make the numbers on your scale fluctuate. And, because muscle weighs more than body fat, when you begin your exercise regime, you might even show a slight weight gain. Not to worry. Remember that the Polar Fat Free and Fit Forever Program is a lifetime regime, a way of healthy living that will be with you always. You don't have to throw your scale away, but it is best used as a secondary indicator of your progress. Use your scale only once a week to see if you are losing your unwanted pound or two or, once you've reached your goal, to see if you are maintaining your new weight.

fact that lean muscle is more dense than fat and tends to sink while the less dense fat tends to float.

Skinfold measurements is another laboratory procedure. Here, the skin is pinched and an instrument called a caliper estimates the fat beneath the skin.

Obviously, these two tests require specialized equipment and trained personnel. However, there is a test you can perform at home which will give you a measurement which correlates very well with body fat. It's called the "body mass index," or BMI. Although it doesn't actually distinguish body fat and muscle, the BMI does correlate with body fat to a high degree.

To determine your BMI based on your height and weight, use the chart on the next page.

To help in your "body fat benchmark" as you lose weight on the Polar Program, I'd also like you to measure the circumference of your waist, abdomen, buttocks, and the middle of your thigh with a simple tape measure. As you begin to lose fat and tone your muscles, you will notice that these circumferences begin to change for the better. Use these tips for accurate measurement (taken from *The Exercise Exchange Program* by Dr. James M. Rippe, New York: Simon & Schuster, 1992):

■ **The Waist.** To find your natural waistline, look in the mirror and find the narrowest spot just below your rib cage. Place the tape measure around your waist so it's slightly taut.

■ **The Abdomen.** Place the tape measure directly over your belly button and draw the tape around your abdomen, making sure it's even.

■ **The Buttocks.** Look in the mirror to find the widest section of your buttocks. Place the tape around you at that spot, making sure it's even and hasn't slipped up or down.

■ **The Middle of the Thigh.** This is the hardest one to locate. To find the correct spot, place the tape measure at the crease at the top of the thigh, directly in line with the hip bone. Then extend the tape down to the kneecap. Mark the part of the thigh that's at the halfway point of the tape. This is the section of thigh you should measure.

Record your BMI and your circumference measurements in the "Vital Statistics" chart found in the Appendix. When you take this test again at ten weeks and at twenty weeks into the Polar program, you'll be able to see how your numbers have shrunk as a result of your good work!

THE POLAR FAT TEST

Over consumption of fat combined with an inactive lifestyle makes for obesity. And, unfortunately, as most of us know by now, there is far too much fat in the American diet. The Polar Fat Free and Fit Forever Program is based on healthy eating.

The BMI Nomogram

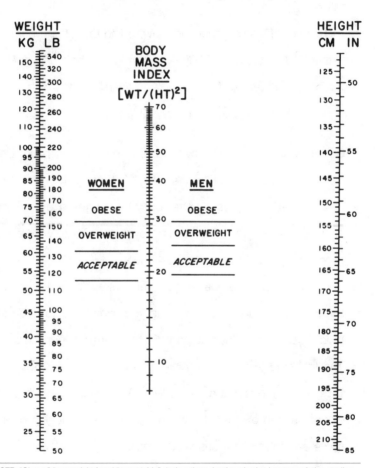

NOTE: "Obese," "overweight,' and "acceptable" designations developed using large population studies.

A nomogram for determining body mass index (BMI). To use this nomogram, place a ruler or other straight edge between the column for height and the column for weight connecting an individual's numbers for those two variables. Read the BMI in kg/m² where the straight line crosses the middle lines when the height and weight are connected. *Overweight:* BMI of 24 to 30 kg/m² ; *Obesity:* BMI above kg/m². Heights and weights are without shoes or clothes.

To that end, it's important to understand and recognize the fats in your diet. Some are easy to spot: butter, salad dressings, sour cream, margarine, and more. High-fat foods are also easy: potato chips, French fries, ice cream — the list, as we all know, can go on . . . and on. But some fats are hidden and harder to recognize. In fact, studies show that 60 percent of the fat in our diet is hidden. And it's these hidden fats that can sabotage the best diet intentions.

Test your fat savvy and learn how to find the fats in your diet with this "Fat Detective" quiz (taken from *The Rockport Walking Program* by Dr. James M. Rippe, Ann Ward, Ph.D., with Karla Dougherty, New York: Fireside Press, 1989):

1. Complete the blank one-day food diary on the next page. Use the format used on the "obvious fat," "fat incognito," and "fats undercover" samples on the following pages. Remember: There's no cheating. This is for your eyes only. Try to write down everything you eat during these 24 hours.

2. You're now ready to analyze your fat intake. You will be going through your diary three times as you examine it for high-fat foods. Use the Fat Chart on page 66 to determine your score.

3. The first time through your diary, you are looking for **obvious fats** — the foods that are virtually 100 percent fat and that are easy to see in our diet. Butter, margarine, and cooking oil are some examples of obvious fats. When you spot an obvious fat in your diary, circle both the food item and the amount that was used. (Refer to the Sample Food Diary of Obvious Fats on page 63.) Compare the amount you used with the amounts on the Fat

Blank Food Diary for
Fat Detective Quiz

H = Home
R = Restaurant (please specify)
C = Cafeteria
O = Other (please specify)

Name: _____
Date Food Consumed: _____

Time	Place	Food Item: Description	Quantity

(NOTE: Diary taken from The Rockport Walking Program by Dr. James M. Rippe, Ann Ward, Ph.D., with Karla Dougherty, New York: Fireside Press, 1989.)

Chart. Keep track of how many "pats" you are using on a separate piece of paper.

4. The second time around, you are looking for **fats incognito.** These are foods that are naturally high in fat. More than 50% of their calories come from fat, but we're not always aware of this because we can't see the fat. Fats incognito include olives, sour cream, and frankfurters. Again, circle all of the foods on your diary that fit this description and jot down how many "pats" you had in your diet.

5. The third and final time through your food diary you're looking for **fats undercover.** Like fats incognito, these are fats we cannot see but have been added during the preparation of food and have made the end result high in fat. Muffins, gravy, french fries, and cookies are examples of fats undercover. Follow the same procedure as with the other fats to record how many "pats" you had.

6. Add up your three "pat" scores. You now have a total number of "pats" for the day, indicating the number of teaspoons of fat that were consumed for that day. Here are some guidelines you can follow to help you better understand what your total number means:

■ If you were eating a **1,200-calorie** diet with 30 percent fat (American Heart Association recommendation), you would not want to exceed eight pats of fat per day.

■ If you were following a **1,500-calorie** diet with 30 percent fat, you would be limited to ten pats of fat per day.

■ If you were following an **1,800-calorie** diet with 30 percent fat, you would be eating no more than 12 pats of fat per day.

Sample Food Diary Showing Obvious Fats

Obvious Fats

- ■ butter (2 tsp.) = 2 pats
- ■ mayonnaise (2 tsp.) = 2 pats

Total = 4 pats

FOOD DIARY

PRE
DIET

Name: John Diary
Date Food Consumed: Mon. January 1, 1991

H = Home
R = Restaurant (please specify)
C = Cafeteria
O = Other (please specify)

Time	Place	Food Item: Description	Quantity
8:00	H	wheat toast with (butter)	2 slices/(2tsp. butter)
		Cheerios with milk (whole)	2 cups/1 cup milk
		orange juice	6 oz.
		coffee with cream	8 oz. coffee/1 tbsp. cream
10:00	O	bran muffin with butter	1 large/2 tsp. butter
	office desk	decaf coffee with cream (half + half)	8 oz. coffee/1 tbsp. cream
1:00	C	ham + cheese sandwich on bulky roll	2 oz ham/1oz Am. cheese
		(mayonnaise)	(2 tsp.)
		potato chips	25 chips
		tossed salad (iceberg lettuce, onions, carrots, cukes)	2 cups
		italian dressing	2 tbsp.
		cherry pie	1/8 of pie
		milk (whole)	12 oz.
3:00	O	delicious apple	1 large
	break room	can of coke	12 oz.
7:00	R	extra crispy thigh + breast	1 of each
	Kentucky Fried Chicken	cole slaw	1 serving
		mashed potato with gravy	1 serving/1 tbsp
		biscuit with butter	1 pat butter/1 medium
		Sprite	medium-15 oz.
9:00	H	mint chocolate chip ice cream (Hood)	3 scoops/1½ cups

(NOTE: Sample diary taken from *The Rockport Walking Program* by Dr. James M. Rippe, Ann Ward, Ph.D., with Karla Dougherty, New York: Fireside Press, 1989.)

Sample Food Diary Showing Fats Incognito

FOOD DIARY

H = Home
R = Restaurant (please specify)
C = Cafeteria
O = Other (please specify)

Name: _John Diary_
Date Food Consumed: _Mon. January 1, 1989_

Time	Place	Food Item: Description	Quantity
8:00	H	wheat toast with butter	2 slices/2 tsp. butter
		cheerios with milk (whole)	2 cups/1 cup milk
		orange juice	6 oz.
		coffee with cream	8 oz. coffee/1 tbsp. cream
10:00	office	bran muffin with butter	1 large/2 tsp. butter
	desk	decaf coffee with cream (half+half)	8 oz. coffee/1 tbsp. cream
1:00	C	ham + cheese sandwich on bulky roll	2 oz. ham/1 oz. Am.cheese
		mayonnaise	2 tsp.
		potato chips	25 chips
		tossed salad (iceberg lettuce, onions, carrots, cukes)	2 cups
		Italian dressing	2 tbsp.
		cherry pie	1/8 of pie
		milk (whole)	12 oz.
3:00	O	delicious apple	1 large
	break room	can of coke	12 oz.
7:00	R	extra crispy thigh + breast	1 of each
	Kentucky	cole slaw	1 serving
	Fried	mashed potato with gravy	1 serving/1 tbsp.
	Chicken	biscuit with butter	1 pat butter/1 medium
		Sprite	medium - 15 oz.
9:00	H	mint chocolate chip (ice cream) (Hood)	3 scoops (1½ cups)

Fats incognito

- whole milk (20 oz.) = 5 pats
- cream, regular (1 tbsp.) = ½ pat
  half + half (1 tbsp.) = ½ pat (cream)
- Cheese (1 oz.) = 2 pats
- Salad dressing (2 tbsp.) = 3 pats
- ice cream (1½ cups) = 4½ pats

Total = 15½ pats

(NOTE: Sample diary taken from *The Rockport Walking Program* by Dr. James M. Rippe, Ann Ward, Ph.D., with Karla Dougherty, New York: Fireside Press, 1989.)

Sample Food Diary Showing Fats Undercover

FOOD DIARY

Name: _John Diary_

PRE / DIET

H = Home
R = Restaurant (please specify)
C = Cafeteria
O = Other (please specify)

Date Food Consumed: _Mon. January 1, 1991_

Time	Place	Food Item: Description	Quantity
8:00	H	wheat toast with butter	2 slices/2 tsp. butter
		cheerios with milk (whole)	2 cups/1 cup milk
		orange juice	6 oz.
		coffee with cream	8 oz. coffee/1 tbsp. cream
10:00	O	bran muffin with butter	1 large/2 tsp. butter
	office desk	decaf coffee with cream (half + half)	8 oz. coffee/1 tbsp. cream
1:00	C	ham + cheese sandwich on bulky roll	2 oz. ham/1 oz. Am. cheese
		mayonnaise	2 tsp.
		potato chips	25 chips
		tossed salad (iceberg lettuce, onions, carrots, cukes)	2 cups
		italian dressing	2 tbsp.
		cherry pie	1/8 of pie
		milk (whole)	12 oz.
3:00	O break room	delicious apple	1 large
		can of coke	12 oz.
7:00	R Kentucky Fried Chicken	extra crispy thigh + breast	1 of each
		cole slaw	1 serving
		mashed potato with gravy	1 serving/1 tbsp.
		biscuit with butter	1 pat butter/1 medium
		sprite	medium—15 oz.
9:00	H	mint chocolate chip ice cream (Hood)	3 scoops/1½ cups

Fats undercover

- muffin (1 large) = 2 pats
- potato chips (25) = 3½ pats
- fried chicken (1 thigh, 1 breast) = 6 pats
- cole slaw (1 serving) = 1 pat
- gravy (1 tbsp.) = 1 pat
- biscuit (1) = 1 pat

Total = 14½ pats
Grand Total = 34 pats

(NOTE: Sample diary taken from *The Rockport Walking Program* by Dr. James M. Rippe, Ann Ward, Ph.D., with Karla Dougherty, New York: Fireside Press, 1989.)

Fat Chart of Common Foods

	PRODUCT/AMOUNT	PAT(S) OF FAT**
Obvious Fats (100% fat; visible fat)	Butter, 1 Tbsp.	3
	Lard, 1 Tbsp.	3
	Margarine, 1 Tbsp.	3
	Mayonnaise, 1 Tbsp.	2
	Vegetable oil, 1 Tbsp.	3
	Vegetable shortening, 1 Tbsp.	3
Fats Incognito (in general, more than 50% fat; foods that are naturally high in fat; invisible fat)	Cream cheese, 2 Tbsp.	2
	Cheese (most types), 1 oz.	2
	Half & Half, 1 fl. oz.	1
	Ice cream 10% fat (supermarket), 1 cup	3
	Ice cream 16% fat (gourmet), 1 cup	5
	Sour cream, 2 Tbsp.	1
	Table cream, 1 fl. oz.	1
	2% milk, 1 cup	1
	Whipped cream, ¼ cup	2
	Whole milk, 1 cup	2
	Egg, whole, medium	1
	Avocado, ⅓ medium	2
	Nuts, ¼ cup	4
	Olives, 10 medium	1
	Peanut butter, 2 Tbsp.	3
	Salad dressing, 2 Tbsp.	3
	Seeds, 1 oz.	3
	Bacon, 3 slices	2
	Bologna, 1 oz.	2
	Cheeseburger, ¼ lb regular ground beef, cooked	6
	Frankfurter, 1 medium	3
	Hamburger, ¼ lb regular ground beef, cooked	4
	Sausage, 1 oz.	2
	Sirloin steak, 6 oz.	6
	T-bone steak, 6 oz.	8
Fats Undercover (fat added during preparation; invisible fat)	Biscuit, 1 medium	2
	Croissant, 1 medium	2
	Muffin, 1 large	2
	Corn chips/tortilla chips, 1 oz.	2
	Crackers (butter-type), 5	1
	French fries, 1 cup/15, 2″-3″ long	2
	Popcorn, microwave (movie theater), 4 cups	2
	Potato chips, 1 oz./15 chips	2
	Cheese sauce, ¼ cup	2
	Gravy, homemade brown, ¼ cup	3
	White sauce, thick, ¼ cup	2
	Chicken, breaded and fried, 3 oz.	3
	Fish, breaded and fried, 3 oz.	2
	Mayonnaise-based salads (potato/macaroni/coleslaw), ½ cup	2
	Pizza, (15″ diameter), 1 slice	2
	Cookies, chocolate chip (2¼″ diameter), 4	2
	Cookies, oatmeal (2 ⅝″ diameter), 4	2
	Pie, any kind	3

Source: Paula Cuneo, R.D., and Merry Yamartino, R.D.   **1 pat = 1 teaspoon or 5 grams of fat.

(NOTE: Chart taken from *The Rockport Walking Program* by Dr. James M. Rippe, Ann Ward, Ph.D., with Karla Dougherty, New York: Fireside Press, 1989, page 25)

THE POLAR HEART TEST

T he Polar Fat Free and Fit Forever Program is more than a weight loss regimen. It is a program of lifelong health and fitness. Therefore, before embarking on the Polar Fat Free and Fit Forever Program, I strongly recommend you be tested for cholesterol levels and have your blood pressure taken. Both high cholesterol and high blood pressure are major risk factors for coronary disease — and reducing them is a major step towards health. A diet and exercise regime like the Polar Program can help you decrease both elevated cholesterol and high blood pressure. Recording and understanding the results your physician finds can help you stay motivated on your program, especially when you get retested ten and twenty weeks into the Polar Fat Free and Fit Forever Program and the numbers are down! To help your medical motivation, here are two quizzes to test your heart knowledge (taken from *The Rockport Walking Program* by Dr. James M. Rippe, Ann Ward, Ph.D., with Karla Dougherty, New York: Fireside Press, 1989, page 41-43):

■ Evaluating Cholesterol Values ■

Answer True or False to the following statements:

1. Total cholesterol should be measured in every adult 45 years and older.

2. Getting your cholesterol measured every 10 years is a good rule of thumb.

3. A measurement below 200 milligrams per deciliter of blood is a "desirable blood-cholesterol" level.

4. A "borderline-high blood cholesterol" is any measurement between 200 and 239 milligrams per deciliter of blood.

5. "High blood cholesterol" is classified as any measurement above 240 milligrams per deciliter of blood.

6. Men are considered at a higher risk when cholesterol values are measured.

Answers

1. **False.** Adults should start having their cholesterol tested when they reach their twenties.

2. **False.** The National Heart, Lung, and Blood Institute recommends that adults get retested for cholesterol at least every five years.

3. **True.** But that doesn't mean you can forget about the risks of high cholesterol. For the best preventive care, keep your intake of saturated fats low, your exercise program consistent, and do get retested every five years.

4. **True.** If your levels are in the borderline range, we suggest you repeat your blood-cholesterol test to confirm the value. If you do not have coronary heart disease and you don't have more than two other risk factors (see Chapter One), your levels can be controlled by a low-fat diet. But do have a cholesterol test taken once a year. However, if you have two or more coronary heart disease risk factors in addition to your high blood-cholesterol, a lipoprotein analysis should be done to determine your LDL-cholesterol level. Consult your physician for the best course of action.

5. **True.** A lipoprotein analysis is recommended at this point. Medication may or may not be prescribed — depending on

other coronary heart disease risk factors you might have. Consult your physician on drug treatment and dietary guidelines.

6. **True.** In addition to the eight risk factors for coronary heart disease discussed in Chapter One, being male is considered an additional risk.

Scoring

K nowledge is only the first step in preventive care. Whether you've answered all six questions correctly or incorrectly is not the point. The real points are: Eat a healthy, low-fat diet, participate in a consistent exercise program, listen to your physician, and have your cholesterol checked on a regular basis.

■ Understanding Your Blood-Pressure Readings■

See if you can answer the following questions:

1. What do the terms *systolic* and *diastolic* mean?
2. What is a mild high-blood-pressure reading?
3. How can you lower your blood pressure?
4. How often should you have your blood pressure taken?
5. What exactly is *hypertension*?

Answers

1. *Systolic* blood pressure is the upper number of your reading, and it reflects the pressure your heart exerts when it squeezes down and contracts, pushing the blood through your arteries. *Diastolic* blood pressure is the lower number of your reading, and it reflects the pressure the arteries feel while the heart is resting between beats. A high-blood-pressure reading means that the

heart is squeezing too hard to get the blood moving through your arteries (systolic), and the blood in the arteries is straining too hard to flow smoothly and evenly while the heart rests (diastolic).

2. You can be considered as having mild high blood pressure if your reading is above 140/90.

3. High blood pressure can be prevented through a regular program of diet and exercise. Remember, for every two pounds of weight you lose, you'll lose one millimeter of mercury off your blood pressure reading. Our studies at the Exercise Physiology and Nutrition Laboratory have shown that daily aerobic exercise will help reduce your blood pressure — and keep it low. Medication can also help lower blood pressure. Consult your physician for specific guidelines.

4. More than 60 million Americans have high blood pressure — and between 30 and 40 percent of all Americans do not even know what their blood pressure is. Today, getting your blood pressure taken is as accessible as your corner drugstore. We suggest you have your blood pressure taken at least twice a year.

5. *Hypertension* is another name for high blood pressure. It literally means increased *(hyper)* pressure *(tension)*. Hypertension can be inherited, but 90 percent of all cases are a mystery. For some reason — and nobody understands what this reason is — arterial pressure can get elevated and result in hypertension. But high blood pressure can be prevented by a regular program of weight loss and exercise like the Polar Fat Free and Fit Forever Program.

THE POLAR AEROBICS TEST

I n 1986, we introduced the One-Mile Walk Test at the American College of Sports Medicine's annual meeting. Before that time, there was no one simple — and accurate — test that individuals could take at home to estimate their aerobic capacity.

Based on a rigorous scientific study of over 300 people tested at my Exercise Physiology and Nutrition Laboratory and at the Department of Exercise Science at the University of Massachusetts in Amherst, the One-Mile Walk Test has received a great deal of national attention. It has been discussed on such shows as *Today* and *Good Morning, America* and in *USA Today.* Over two million people and organizations have written to us asking for copies of the brochure that describes the test. And most modern exercise physiology texts now feature the test as a good way for individuals to estimate their aerobic capacity.

The One-Mile Walk Test is based on your heart rate response to the simple task of briskly walking a mile. When we first developed the test, we felt it was essential to achieve absolute accuracy in measuring the heart rate in order to achieve scientifically valid information. To that end, we used Polar Heart Rate Monitors on **all** of our research subjects, both to monitor their heart rates and their time to walk the mile. Using your heart rate monitor, you can achieve the same level of accuracy.

By taking this One-Mile Walk Test you will determine how your aerobic capacity compares to other individuals of your age and sex. It will also give you the information you need to determine which of the five exercise programs, Blue (Starter), Green (Beginner), Yellow (Intermediate), Orange (Advanced), or Red (Expert) is the right one for you to follow.

Once you know your program, you can begin the Polar Way in the exercise of your choice.

(If your exercise of choice is Stepping or Lifecycling, there are Stepping and Lifecycle self-tests in the Appendix that you can use to determine your fitness level and exercise program.)

Let's go walking and take the One-Mile Walk Test now! (Test taken from *The Rockport Walking Program* by Dr. James M. Rippe, Ann Ward, Ph.D., with Karla Dougherty, New York: Fireside Press, 1989.)

■ Before You Start:

1. **Determine your heart rate by using the Polar Heart Rate Monitor.** I recommend that individuals use the heart rate monitor to determine resting heart rate as well as their heart rate response to warm-up and stretching simply to get used to the measurement.

2. Find a mile-length track. Since you'll be walking one mile as briskly as you can for the One-Mile Test you need to determine your route before you start. Choose a route that's as flat and smooth as possible. Most high schools, colleges, and local health clubs and recreational facilities have quarter-mile tracks. If you map out one mile with your car's odometer, pick a route with the least amount of stoplights, crowded sidewalks, and traffic.

3. **Warm up and stretch for five minutes.** Warming up helps

get the blood flowing to your muscles. Once you've warmed up, stretching your muscles will keep them from getting stiff. (You'll find warm-up suggestions and stretching exercises in the next chapter.)

■ Taking the Test Step-By-Step:

1. **Walk the mile as briskly as you can.**
2. **At the end of the mile, immediately look at your heart rate monitor to determine your heart rate.**
3. **Record your time to the nearest second.** It should take you somewhere between 10 and 25 minutes to walk the mile. (If you are using the Polar Favor model, you will need to use a watch with a second-hand to determine your time. All other Polar models record time as well as heart rate. See Appendix A on page 143.)
4. **That's it.** You are now ready to find your relative fitness level and the Polar Heart Rate Monitor exercise program that's right for you.

■ Finding Your Fitness Level:

1. **Find the relative fitness graph on pages 76-79 that best fits your age and sex.** Based on fitness norms established by the American Heart Association, it will show how your performance compares with others your age and sex.
2. **Mark the point defined by your One-Mile Walk Test results.** Mark your walking time on the timescale along the

bottom. Mark your heart rate at the end of the walk on the left side of the scale. Draw a vertical line from your walk time and a horizontal line from your heart rate to the point where they intersect. The area where these two points meet shows your relative fitness level: either high, above average, average, below average, or low as compared to others in your age and sex category.

For example, a 42-year-old woman who weighed 180 pounds completed the One-Mile Walk Test in 18 minutes, 15 seconds, and had a heart rate at the end of the mile of 132 beats per minute. Her heart rate line and timeline converged in the below average fitness category.

■ Finding Your Individual Exercise Program:

1. **Find the exercise program on the following pages that best fits your age and sex.** Mark the time and your heart rate just as you did on the relative fitness graph. The labeled area where these two points converge shows you the specific exercise program that is just right for you: either Blue, Green, Yellow, Orange, or Red.

2. **Remember your program name.** In the next chapter, you'll be putting your individual exercise program into practice — with a full twenty week program for each color: Blue, Green, Yellow, Orange, or Green.

   For example, the 42-year-old woman described above fell into the Green Exercise Program Chart and began her Polar Program with the Green 20-week exercise prescription.

3. **Write the time it took to walk the mile as well as your**

heart rate response on your "Vital Statistics" Chart in Appendix B. (page 145) When you repeat the One-Mile Walk Test at 10 and 20 weeks, you'll be amazed at the improvement — and motivated to keep up the good work!

• • • • • • • • •

ongratulations! You've just completed the Polar tests that will provide an initial benchmark for your personal Polar program. You might say that the testing was as easy as one, two, three:

One: Determining your body fat

Two: Learning about hidden fat, blood cholesterol, and blood pressure

Three: Estimating your aerobic capacity

In the next chapter, we're going to use the results of these tests to get you started on your personal, lifelong Polar program. Let's go. . . .

Relative Fitness Levels and Exercise Programs

20–29-Year-Olds

Relative Fitness Levels

Females

Males

Exercise Program

Females

Males

30–39-Year-Olds

Relative Fitness Levels

Females

Males

The charts found on pages 76–79 are taken from *The Exercise Exchange Program* by Dr. James M. Rippe, New York: Simon & Schuster, 1992.

The One Mile Walk Test used with permission of the author: Dr. James M. Rippe.

Exercise Program

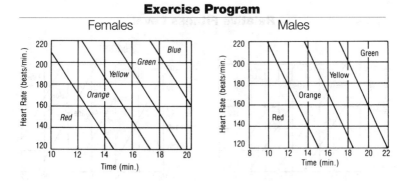

Relative Fitness Level

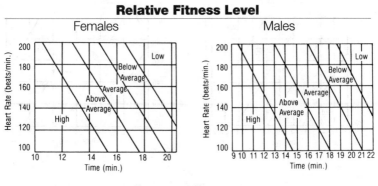

Exercise Program

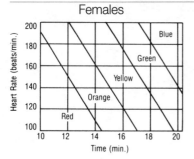
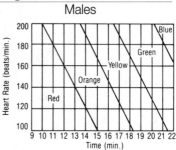

Relative Fitness Level

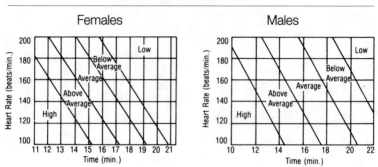

Exercise Program

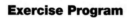

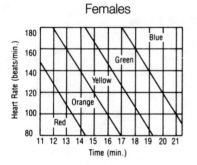

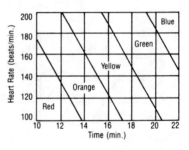

Relative Fitness Level

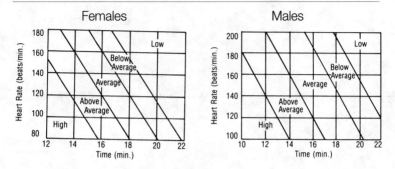

Exercise Program

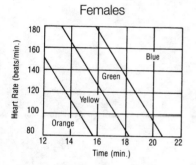
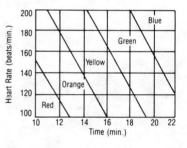

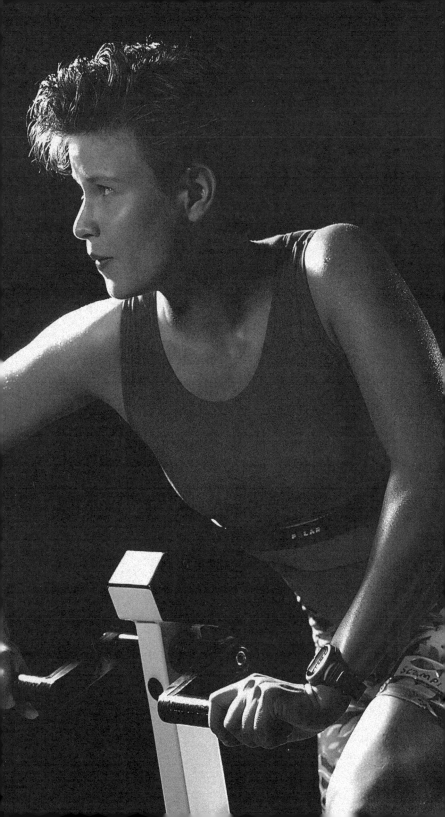

Your Individual Polar Exercise Program

"Three weeks ago, I couldn't even imagine walking to the store,

a distance of about three hundred yards.

Now, thanks to Polar, I'm walking almost two miles

three times a week and I feel great!"

—A 38-year-old manager who'd just started the Polar Fat Free
and Fit Forever Program

You've read through the principles behind the Polar

Fat Free and Fit Forever Program. You've taken the four self-tests
and you now know your own individual ground rules:

■ The amount of body fat you want to lose

■ The fat — obvious, incognito, and undercover — you want to
eliminate from your diet

■ The blood-cholesterol levels and blood pressure readings you want to decrease

■ The fitness level and exercise program that's most effective for you to lose weight without injury on the Polar Fat Free and Fit Forever Program.

In this chapter, we'll get you started on your exercise program. The next chapter will put you on the right nutrition track. Together, you'll have a complete, individualized program that you can start right now.

So, without further ado, here's. . . .

THE POLAR 20-WEEK EXERCISE PROGRAM

By now, you've taken the One-Mile Walk Test, the Lifecycle Fit Test (see appendix), or the STEP Fit Test™ (see appendix), and you've determined which color program is right for you, based on your relative fitness, age, and sex. In this chapter, you will find 20-week programs — and beyond — for the following exercises:

- Walking
- Walk/Jog/Run

- Step Aerobics
- Lifecycle

But before we go on to the actual programs, there are some things you need to know — regardless of which exercise you choose to follow.

STAYING IN YOUR TARGET WEIGHT MANAGEMENT ZONE

For maximum results, we recommend you stay within the Weight Management Zone during your exercise routine. As we have seen in Chapter Two, this is 60-70 percent of your maximum heart rate. (Use the Target Heart Rate Zone table on page 45 for easy reference.) We recommend your starting at 60 percent and working your way up to 70 percent — the higher end of the Weight Management Zone. After ten weeks into your exercise regime, start aiming for the Aerobic Training Zone — between 70 and 80 percent of your maximum heart rate. But don't push yourself too hard. Remember, slow and steady wins the long-term race.

Use your Polar Heart Monitor as your "personal coach." Your Polar Heart Rate Monitor will ensure that you are within the right zone for the best fat-burning workout — without injury. If you see that you are going beyond your target zone, you can ease up. If you aren't reaching your zone, the monitor will show that you need to put more energy into your workout. If your exercise routine is starting to feel too "easy," move towards the higher end (70 percent) of your Weight Management Zone. Use your monitor to move into the Aerobic Training Zone when you've completed your 10 weeks — and use it to go back a few percentages if you're feeling any pain or over exhaustion. Let your Polar Heart Monitor be the judge, pushing you forward or moving you back, higher or lower, for the best possible **personal** workout without injury.

WARM-UPS AND COOL-DOWNS

Whatever the exercise, I highly recommend five minutes of warm-up before you begin your routine and five minutes of cool-down when you finish.

Warming up gives your body a chance to literally "rev up." Doing the exercise of your choice at a leisurely rate will loosen muscles and aid flexibility, helping you avoid soreness, muscle pulls, or injury. Warming up will also help you avoid unnecessary cardiac strain. You can use your Polar Heart Rate Monitor to see how your heart is responding to your warm-up; you can use your monitor to make sure you don't "rev up" to your Weight Management Zone too quickly.

Cooling down helps you "come down" from your target heart rate zone, helping you avoid undo strain on your heart. Cooling down can also help prevent muscle soreness and keep your flexibility up.

STRETCHING

I also recommend stretching after you've warmed up or cooled down for about three to four minutes. Stretching is different from a warm-up or a cool-down — and **you should never do your stretches before you've had a chance to warm your body up.** Stretching relieves stress and increases your flexibility and sense of well-being all day long.

The best time to stretch is after you've warmed up in the exercise of your choice. The following exercises are a series of simple stretches that you can do after a warm-up or before a cool-down.

Perform these stretches slowly and smoothly until you feel a slight "tugging" sensation on the muscles involved. But don't stretch to the point you feel pain — and don't bounce; you might pull a muscle. Hold each stretch for 10 to 15 seconds. (These stretches are taken from *The Rockport Walking Program* by Dr. James M. Rippe, Ann Ward, Ph.D., with Karla Dougherty, New York: Fireside Press, 1989, page 57-59).

1. Calf (back of lower leg)

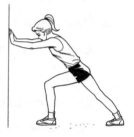

a. Straight knee — start with the leg to be stretched approximately three feet from the wall and the opposite leg one step forward. Lean toward wall, keeping heels down and foot turned in slightly.

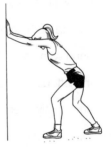

b. Bent knee — start same as above, but move approximately one foot closer to the wall and bend knee of back leg to be stretched.

c. Repeat using other leg.

2. Iliotibial Band (outside of hip)

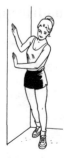

a. Start with leg to be stretched one step back and behind opposite foot. Move hips sideways toward side being stretched. Keep upper body away from wall and do not bend forward.

b. Repeat using other leg.

3. Lower Back, Hips, Groin, and Hamstrings

Stand with feet about shoulder-width apart and pointed straight ahead. Slowly bend forward from the hips. Always keep knees slightly bent. Go to the point where you feel a slight stretch in the back of your legs.

4. Side Bends

a. Stand with your feet about shoulder-width apart and toes pointed straight ahead. Keep your knees slightly bent, one hand on your hip; extend your other arm up and over your head. Slowly bend at your waist to the side, toward the hand on your hip.

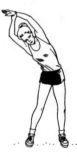

b. Extend both arms overhead. Hold your right hand with your left hand and bend slowly to the left, using your left arm to pull the right arm gently over the head and down toward the ground.

c. Repeat with other side.

5. Quadriceps (front of thigh)

a. Lying on your stomach, pull heel toward buttocks with opposite hand. Keep thigh in close to other leg.

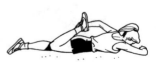

b. The same stretch can be done standing. Do not allow thigh to come in front of you and do not bend forward at the waist.

c. Do this exercise twice — once for each leg.

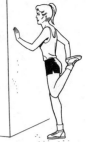

6. Groin (inside of thigh)

a. Sit on floor with soles of feet together. Gently push knees down toward floor with elbows.

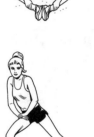

b. Stand with feet three to four feet apart and turned out slightly. Keep knee of leg to be stretched straight, and bend opposite knee as you move your body toward the bent leg. Keep toes pointed forward.

c. Repeat using other leg.

7. Hamstrings (back of thigh)

a. Sit with one knee bent and leg to be stretched out straight. Reach for toes of straight leg with right hand and then left hand.

b. Repeat with other leg.

8. Gluteus (back of hip)

a. Lie on your back. Pull one knee up to chest while keeping opposite leg down on the floor with knee straight.

b. The same may be done standing.

c. Repeat with other leg.

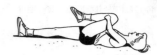

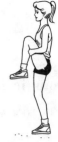

9. Anterior Tibialis (front of shin)

a. Stand with all of your weight on one leg. Extend opposite leg forward and flex and point at the ankle.

b. Repeat using the other leg.

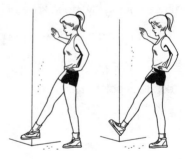

YOUR 20-WEEK PROGRAM

You've warmed up for five minutes. You've done your three minutes of stretches. You're limber, loose, and ready to go. Here's the program you will follow for the next 20 weeks — and beyond. Find the exercise of your choice on the following pages, look for the color that corresponds to the color you're to follow based on your self-test results, and, as the commercial says, "Just Do It!"

20-WEEK FITNESS STEPPING PROGRAM

The basic stepping movements include:

■ Basic Right: Right leg leads. Right foot up on Step platform, left foot up on platform, right foot down on floor, then left.

■ Basic Left: Left leg leads. Left foot up on Step, right foot up on Step, left foot down on floor, then right.

■ March on floor. March in place next to Step platform.

■ Pump arms. Start with arms at side, relaxed. Then begin to pump arms in time with steps.

Each program gives you the step height you should work with, the cadence (pace) of your steps per minute, the time you need to exercise, and how many times each week you need to do your step aerobics. At the end of your first 10 weeks, retest yourself and begin the next 10 weeks — most likely at another level!

BLUE

WARM-UP[1]	4 minutes
STEP HEIGHT	4 inches
CADENCE	116 counts per minute
FREQUENCY	3-4 x per week
Week 1-2	12 minutes
Week 3-4	16 minutes
Week 5-7	20 minutes
Week 8-10	24 minutes
Retest	
MOVEMENTS	1 minute basic-Right
	1 minute march on floor
	1 minute basic-Left
	1 minute march on floor
	Repeat
COOL-DOWN[2]	4 minutes

GREEN

WARM-UP[1]	4 minutes
STEP HEIGHT	4 inches
CADENCE	116 counts per minute
FREQUENCY	3-4 x per week
Week 1-2	12 minutes
Week 3-4	16 minutes
Week 5-7	20 minutes
Week 8-10	24 minutes
Retest	
MOVEMENTS	1 minute basic-Right
	1 minute basic-Left
	Repeat
COOL-DOWN[2]	4 minutes

YELLOW

WARM-UP[1]	4 minutes
STEP HEIGHT	6 inches
CADENCE	116 counts per minute
FREQUENCY	3-4 x per week
Week 1-2	12 minutes
Week 3-4	16 minutes
Week 5-7	20 minutes
Week 8-10	24 minutes
Retest	
MOVEMENTS	1 minute basic-Right
	1 minute basic-Left
	Repeat
COOL-DOWN[2]	4 minutes

ORANGE

WARM-UP[1]	4 minutes
STEP HEIGHT	8 inches[3]
CADENCE	124 counts per minute
FREQUENCY	3-4 x per week
Week 1-3	16 minutes
Week 4-7	20 minutes
Week 8-10	24 minutes
Retest	
MOVEMENTS	1 minute basic-Right
	1 minute basic-Left
	Pump arms
	Repeat
COOL-DOWN[2]	4 minutes

RED

WARM-UP[1]	4 minutes
STEP HEIGHT	8 inches[3]
CADENCE	124 counts per minute
FREQUENCY	3-4 x per week
Week 1-3	16 minutes
Week 4-7	20 minutes
Week 8-10	24 minutes
Retest	
MOVEMENTS	1 minute basic-Right
	1 minute basic-Left
	Alternate knee lifts to finish
	Pump arms
COOL-DOWN[2]	4 minutes

(1) warm-up consists of marching in place plus stretching
(2) Cool-down same as warm-up
(3) If not currently Step Training, use 6" STEP for weeks 1–3 of program.

20-Week Walking Program

The left-side of this chart tells you how fast you need to walk (pace), how long it should take, the mileage you need to cover, how long it should take, the number of calories you will burn with each workout, and how many days a week you need to walk. Across the top, you'll find the weeks of your program, from one to 20 and beyond (for either moving ahead or maintaining your new-found weight loss and fitness level.)

Twenty-Week Walking Program*

Program	Weeks	1	2	3-4	5-6	7-8	9-10	11-12	13-14	15-16	17-18	19-20	Progression or Maintenance
BLUE	Pace	3.0	3.0	3.0	3.25	3.5	3.5	3.75	3.75	3.75	4.0	4.0	Go to Green, week 15
	Minutes	22.0	22.0	27.0	26.0	29.0	29.0	28.0	28.0	34.0	34.0	34.0	
	Mileage	1.1	1.1	1.4	1.4	1.7	1.7	1.8	1.8	2.1	2.2	2.2	
	Calories	86.0	86.0	108.0	113.0	136.0	136.0	145.0	145.0	177.0	196.0	196.0	
	Days/week	3	4	4	5	5	5	5	5	5	5	5	
GREEN	Pace	3.0	3.0	3.0	3.5	3.5	3.5	3.5	4.0	4.0	4.0	4.0	Go to Yellow, week 17, or add hills, light hand weights
	Minutes	25.0	25.0	31.0	28.0	31.0	31.0	34.0	27.0	33.0	39.0	39.0	
	Mileage	1.3	1.3	1.6	1.6	1.8	1.8	2.0	1.8	2.2	2.6	2.6	
	Calories	97.0	97.0	121.0	131.0	147.0	147.0	159.0	159.0	194.0	227.0	227.0	
	Days/week	4	4	5	5	5	5	5	5	5	5	5	
YELLOW	Pace	3.0	3.0	3.0	3.25	3.5	3.5	4.0	4.0	4.0	4.5	4.5	Go to Orange, week 19, or add hills, light hand weights
	Minutes	27.0	33.0	40.0	37.0	37.0	37.0	29.0	32.0	38.0	33.0	36.0	
	Mileage	1.4	1.7	2.0	2.0	2.1	2.1	1.9	2.1	2.5	2.5	2.7	
	Calories	106.0	132.0	159.0	159.0	171.0	171.0	171.0	183.0	223.0	240.0	262.0	
	Days/week	4	5	5	5	5	5	5	5	5	5	5	
ORANGE	Pace	3.5	3.5	3.5	3.75	4.0	4.0	4.0	4.0	4.5	4.5	4.5	Go to Red, week 19, or add hills, light hand weights
	Minutes	26.0	33.0	39.0	35.0	34.0	34.0	34.0	36.0	29.0	31.0	42.0	
	Mileage	1.5	1.9	2.3	2.2	2.2	2.2	2.2	2.4	2.2	2.3	3.1	
	Calories	122.0	152.0	183.0	183.0	197.0	197.0	197.0	210.0	210.0	224.0	298.0	
	Days/week	5	5	5	5	5	5	5	5	4-5	4-5	4-5	
RED	Pace	4.0	4.0	4.0	4.5	4.5	4.5	4.5	4.5	4.5	4.5	4.5	Add hills, light hand weights
	Minutes	24.0	30.0	36.0	29.0	31.0	31.0	31.0	21.0	31.0	32.0	43.0	
	Mileage	1.6	2.0	2.4	2.2	2.3	2.3	2.3	2.3	2.3	2.4	3.2	
	Calories	140.0	175.0	210.0	210.0	224.0	224.0	224.0	224.0	224.0	235.0	313.0	
	Days/week	5	5	5	5	5	5	4-5	4-5	4-5	3-5	3-6	

*Adapted from James M. Rippe and Ann Ward, "Rockport's Guide to Fitness Walking," p. 221. Dr. James M. Rippe's Complete Book of Fitness Walking (New York: Prentice Hall Press, 1989), p. 25-41.

HEART RATE RANGE, ALL GROUPS: Weeks 1-10, 60-70 percent maximum; weeks 11-20, 70-80 percent maximum caloric expenditure based on 154 pound person. To determine your caloric expenditure, add or subtract 10 percent for every 15 pounds above or below 154 pounds. If you are in between, round to the nearer weight range.
Example: If you weigh 169 lbs. and are beginning the Blue level, multiply 86 calories by 10 percent ($86 \times .10 = 8.6$) and add 8.6 to 86 ($86 + 8.6 = 94.6$). Your caloric expenditure for weeks 1-2, Blue, would be approximately 95 calories.

(Chart taken from *The Exercise Exchange Program* by Dr. James M. Rippe, New York: Simon & Schuster, 1992, p.159)

20-Week Walk/Jog/Run Program

Each program shows you the mileage you need to cover, the pace you need to keep (minutes per mile), the time you need to exercise, the number of calories you will burn with each workout, and how many times each week you need to jog.

BLUE Program

Week	Exercise	Mileage	Pace* (mph)	Heart rate (% of max.)	Duration of workout (min.)	Calories burned†	Frequency (times/wk.)
1	Fitness walk	1.00	3.0	60	20	100	3
2	Fitness walk	1.00	3.0	60	20	100	3
3	Fitness walk	1.25	3.0	60	25	125	3
4	Fitness walk	1.25	3.0	60	25	125	3
5	Fitness walk	1.50	3.0	60	30	150	3
6	Fitness walk	1.50	3.5	65–70	26	150	3
7	Fitness walk	1.75	3.5	65–70	30	175	3
8	Fitness walk	1.75	3.5	65–70	30	175	3
9	Fitness walk	2.00	3.5	65–70	34	200	3
10	Fitness walk	2.00	3.75	65–70	32	200	3
11	Fitness walk	2.00	3.75	70–75	32	200	3
12	Fitness walk	2.25	3.75	70–75	36	225	3
13	Fitness walk	2.25	3.75	70–75	36	225	3
14	Fitness walk	2.50	3.75	70–75	40	250	3
15	Fitness walk	2.50	4.0	70–75	38	250	3
16	Fitness walk	2.50	4.0	70–75	38	250	3
17	Fitness walk	2.75	4.0	75–80	41	275	3
18	Fitness walk	2.75	4.0	75–80	41	275	3
19	Fitness walk	2.75	4.0	75–80	41	275	3
20	Fitness walk	2.75	4.0	75–80	41	275	3

*The pace listed is only an approximation. The actual pace to be used is the one that keeps the heart rate at the appropriate % of max.

†Calorie expenditure is for an average 150-pound person. The number of calories burned will be slightly lower for lower body weight and slightly higher for higher body weight.

(Charts taken from *The Sports Performance Factors* by James M. Rippe, M.D., and William Southmayd, M.D., New York: Perigee Books, 1986, p.70-74. Charts reprinted with permission.)

Walk/Jog/Run
GREEN Program

Week	Exercise	Mileage	Pace* (mph)	Heart rate (% of max.)	Duration of workout (min.)	Calories burned†	Frequency (times/wk.)
1	Fitness walk	1.50	3.0	60–65	30	150	3
2	Fitness walk	1.50	3.0	60–65	30	150	3
3	Fitness walk	1.75	3.0	60–65	35	175	3
4	Fitness walk	1.75	3.0	60–65	35	175	3
5	Fitness walk	2.00	3.0	60–65	40	200	3
6	Fitness walk	2.00	3.0	60–65	40	200	3
7	Fitness walk	2.00	3.5	65–70	34	200	3
8	Fitness walk	2.25	3.5	65–70	38	225	3
9	Fitness walk	2.25	3.5	65–70	38	225	3
10	Fitness walk	2.50	3.5	65–70	43	250	3
11	Fitness walk	2.50	3.5	65–70	43	250	3
12	Fitness walk	2.50	3.5	65–70	43	250	3
13	Fitness walk	2.75	3.5	65–70	47	275	3
14	Fitness walk	2.75	3.5	65–70	47	275	3
15	Fitness walk	3.00	4.0	70–80	45	300	3
16	Fitness walk	3.00	4.0	70–80	45	300	3
17	Fitness walk	3.00	4.0	70–80	45	300	3
18	Fitness walk	3.00	4.0	70–80	45	300	3
19	Fitness walk	3.00	4.0	70–80	45	300	3
20	Fitness walk	3.00	4.0	70–80	45	300	3

*The pace listed is only an approximation. The actual pace to be used is the one that keeps the heart rate at the appropriate % of max.
†Calorie expenditure is for an average 150-pound person. The number of calories burned will be slightly lower for lower body weight and slightly higher for higher body weight.

YELLOW Program

Week	Exercise	Mileage	Pace* (mph)	Heart rate (% of max.)	Duration of workout (min.)	Calories burned†	Frequency (times/wk.)
1	Fitness walk	2.00	3.0	65–70	40	200	3
2	Fitness walk	2.25	3.0	65–70	45	225	3
3	Fitness walk	2.50	3.0	65–70	50	250	3
4	Fitness walk	2.50	3.0	65–70	50	250	3
5	Fitness walk	2.75	3.0	65–70	50	275	3
6	Fitness walk	2.75	3.5	70–75	47	275	3
7	Fitness walk	2.75	3.5	70–75	47	275	3
8	Fitness walk	2.75	3.5	70–75	47	275	3
9	Fitness walk	3.00	3.5	70–75	51	300	3
10	Fitness walk	3.00	3.5	70–75	51	300	3
11	Fitness walk	3.00	4.0	75–80	45	300	3
12	Fitness walk	3.00	4.0	75–80	45	300	3
13	Fitness walk	3.25	4.0	75–80	49	325	3
14	Fitness walk	3.25	4.0	75–80	49	325	3
15	Fitness walk	3.50	4.0	75–80	53	350	3
16	Fitness walk	3.50	4.5	75–80	47	350	3
17	Fitness walk	3.50	4.5	75–80	47	350	3
18	Fitness walk	3.50	4.5	75–80	47	350	3
19	Fitness walk	3.50	4.5	75–80	47	350	3
20	Fitness walk	3.50	4.5	75–80	47	350	3

*The pace listed is only an approximation. The actual pace to be used is the one that keeps the heart rate at the appropriate % of max.
†Calorie expenditure is for an average 150-pound person. The number of calories burned will be slightly lower for lower body weight and slightly higher for higher body weight.

Walk/Jog/Run
ORANGE Program

Week	Exercise	Mileage	Pace* (min./ mile)	Heart rate (% of max.)	Duration of workout (min.)	Calories burned†	Frequency (times/wk.)
1	Jog/Run	2.00	8–10	70–75	16–20	200	3
2	Jog/Run	2.00	8–10	70–75	16–20	200	3
3	Jog/Run	2.25	8–10	70–75	18–23	225	3
4	Jog/Run	2.25	8–10	70–75	18–23	225	3
5	Jog/Run	2.50	8–10	70–75	20–25	250	3
6	Jog/Run	2.50	8–10	70–75	20–25	250	3
7	Jog/Run	3.00	8–10	70–75	24–30	300	3
8	Jog/Run	3.50	8–10	75–80	28–35	350	3
9	Jog/Run	3.50	7–10	75–80	25–35	350	3
10	Jog/Run	3.50	7–10	75–80	25–35	350	3
11	Jog/Run	4.00	7–10	75–80	28–40	400	3
12	Jog/Run	4.00	7–10	75–80	28–40	400	3
13	Jog/Run	4.00	7–10	75–80	28–40	400	3
14	Jog/Run	4.00	7–10	75–80	28–40	400	3
15	Jog/Run	4.50	7–10	75–80	28–40	450	3
16	Jog/Run	4.50	7–10	75–80	28–40	450	3
17	Jog/Run	4.50	7–10	75–80	28–40	450	3
18	Jog/Run	5.00	7–10	75–80	28–40	500	3
19	Jog/Run	5.00	7–10	75–80	28–40	500	3
20	Jog/Run	5.00	7–10	75–80	28–40	500	3

*Pace should be determined by the running speed that keeps the heart rate at 70–80% of predicted maximum.
†Calorie expenditure is for an average 150-pound person. The number of calories burned will be slightly lower for lower body weight and slightly higher for higher body weight.

RED Program

Week	Exercise	Mileage	Pace* (min./ mile)	Heart rate (% of max.)	Duration of workout (min.)	Calories burned†	Frequency (times/wk.)
1	Jog/Run	3.00	8–10	75–80	24–30	300	3
2	Jog/Run	3.00	8–10	75–80	24–30	300	3
3	Jog/Run	3.50	8–10	75–80	28–35	350	3
4	Jog/Run	4.00	8–10	75–80	32–40	400	3
5	Jog/Run	4.00	7–10	75–80	28–40	400	3
6	Jog/Run	4.00	7–10	75–80	28–40	400	3
7	Jog/Run	4.50	7–10	75–80	31–45	450	3
8	Jog/Run	4.50	7–10	75–80	31–45	450	3
9	Jog/Run	4.50	7–10	75–80	31–45	450	3
10	Jog/Run	5.00	7–10	75–80	35–50	500	3
11	Jog/Run	5.00	7–10	75–80	35–50	500	3
12	Jog/Run	5.00	7–10	75–80	35–50	500	3
13	Jog/Run	5.50	7–10	75–80	38–55	550	3
14	Jog/Run	5.50	7–10	75–80	38–55	550	3
15	Jog/Run	5.50	7–10	75–80	38–55	550	3
16	Jog/Run	6.00	7–10	75–80	42–60	600	3
17	Jog/Run	6.00	7–10	75–80	42–60	600	3
18	Jog/Run	6.00	7–10	75–80	42–60	600	3
19	Jog/Run	6.00	7–10	75–80	42–60	600	3
20	Jog/Run	6.00	7–10	75–80	42–60	600	3

*Pace should be determined by the running speed that keeps the heart rate at 70–80% of predicted maximum.
†Calorie expenditure is for an average 150-pound person. The number of calories burned will be slightly lower for lower body weight and slightly higher for higher body weight.

20-Week Lifecycle Program

The left-hand side shows you at which level to exercise, the time you need to exercise, the number of calories you will burn with each workout, and how many times each week you need to cycle. Across the top, you'll find the weeks of your program, from one to 20 and beyond (for either moving ahead or maintaining your new-found weight loss and fitness level.)

(Hill Profile)*

Program	Weeks	1	2	3-4	5-6	7-8	9-10	11-12	13-14	15-16	17-18	19-20	Progression or Maintenance
PURPLE	Level	1	1	1	1	2	2	2	2	2	2	3	Go to Blue, week 15
	Minutes	4+4+4	6+6	12	12+3	12+3	12+6	18	18+3	18+6	24	12+12	
	Calories	83	83	83	104	104	129	129	151	173	173	181	
	Days/week	3	3	4	4	4	5	5	5	5	5	5	
BLUE	Level	2	2	2	3	3	3	4	4	4	5	5	Go to Green, week 15
	Minutes	12	12	12+3	12+3	12+6	18	18	18	18+4	12+12	24	
	Calories	86	86	108	113	136	136	145	145	177	196	196	
	Days/week	4	4	4	5	5	5	5	5	5	5	5	
GREEN	Level	4	4	4	5	5	5	6	6	6	7	7	Go to Yellow, week 15
	Minutes	12	12	12+3	12+4	12+6	18	12+6	18	18+4	12+12	24	
	Calories	97	97	121	131	147	147	159	159	194	227	227	
	Days/week	4	4	5	5	5	5	5	5	5	5	5	
YELLOW	Level	6	6	6	6	7	7	7	8	8	9	9	Maintain or go to Orange, week 15
	Minutes	12	12	12+6	18	12+6	18	18	12+6	18+4	18+4	18+6	
	Calories	106	132	159	159	171	171	171	183	223	240	262	
	Days/week	4	5	5	5	5	5	5	5	5	5	5	
ORANGE	Level	8	8	8	8	9	9	9	10	10	11	11	Maintain or go to Red, week 15
	Minutes	12	12+3	12+6	18	12+6	18	18	12+6	18	18	18+6	
	Calories	122	152	183	183	197	197	197	210	210	224	298	
	Days/week	5	5	5	5	5	5	5	5	4-5	4-5	4-5	
RED	Level	10	10	10	10	11	11	11	11	12	12	12	Maintain or cross-train
	Minutes	12	12+3	12+6	18	12+6	12+6	18	18	12+6	18	18+6	
	Calories	140	175	210	210	224	224	224	224	235	235	313	
	Days/week	5	5	5	5	5	5	4-5	4-5	4-5	3-5	3-5	

*Adapted from Rippe, James, and Ward, Ann. *Starting and Staying with Exercise*, brochure by Life Fitness, Inc., 1989. HEART RATE RANGE. ALL GROUPS: Weeks 1–10, 60–70 percent maximum; weeks 11–20, 70–80 percent maximum caloric expenditure based on 154-pound person. To determine your caloric expenditure, add or subtract 10 percent for every 15 pounds above or below 154 pounds. If you are in between, round to the nearer weight range. Example: if you weigh 169 pounds and are beginning the purple level, multiply 83 calories by 10 percent (83 × 10 = 8.3) and add 8.3 to 83 (83 + 8.3 = 91.3). Your caloric expenditure for weeks 1–4, Purple, and level 1, would be approximately 91 calories.

(Chart taken from *The Exercise Exchange Program* by Dr. James M. Rippe, New York: Simon & Schuster, 1992, p.160)

* Note that the Lifecycle program has six colors instead of the usual five. This corresponds to the Lifecycle Self-Test.

STRENGTH TRAINING

I n our research, we've found that the optimal exercise for permanent weight management is a combination of both aerobic exercise and regular resistance strength training. Strength training will make you stronger and more capable of performing your daily routines. It's also the only way I know to increase your lean muscle tissue. In fact, the American College of Sports Medicine now recommends regular high repetition, low-weight strength training as a health promoting measure for all adults.

An excellent way to add strength training to your regular exercise regime is to join a health club or recreational facility. They have the equipment and the instructors to make sure you are training correctly and effectively — with minimal risk of injury.

If you don't have access to a health club, you can perform simple strength training exercises at home. Here are some that we have found to be very successful (taken from *The Exercise Exchange Program* by Dr. James M. Rippe, New York: Simon & Schuster, 1992, p. 364-367):

1. **Half curl-up.** Lie on your back, knees bent, feet close to buttocks. Cross your arms over your chest. Slowly curl your body forward, lifting your head, neck, shoulders, and upper back off the floor. Your lower back should remain flat, in contact with the floor. Then, in a smooth, slow motion, lower your body back down to the floor. One curl should take four seconds (two to curl up, two to lower). For the stomach and upper back.

2. **Alternating knee touch.** Lie on your back, hands behind head, fingers interlocked, elbows out. Now bend your knees and lift them so the lower portion of both legs are resting on a chair or bench. Keeping your lower back on the floor, slowly curl your upper body forward and rotate your trunk so your right elbow touches the left

knee and vice versa. If you can't quite reach your knee with your elbow, move your knee in slightly so your elbow can reach it, allowing you to complete the exercise. For the waist and the stomach.

3. **Double flutter.** Lie on your stomach, hands resting comfortably under your chin, legs straight and together. Tighten your buttocks and slowly lift both feet two to six inches off the ground, then lower your feet slowly. For buttocks and thighs.

4. **Chest raise.** Lie on your stomach, hands behind head, fingers interlocked. Keeping your feet on the ground, slowly lift your head and upper body up from the floor. Hold for two seconds, and return to the ground slowly. If you can't do this alone, ask a partner to hold your feet down. For the lower back, buttocks, and hamstrings.

5. **Push-ups.** Do the same push-ups you did for the push-up test earlier in this section. For the arms, shoulders, and chest.

6. **Inverted push-ups.** Sit with your legs stretched out in front of you. Your palms are flat on the floor behind you, your arms are placed shoulder-width apart. Now raise yourself until your elbows are nearly straight but not locked, your legs are outstretched, and your toes are pointed. Lower yourself until your buttocks just touch the floor, and repeat. For the arms, shoulders, and upper back.

7. **Lunges.** Begin in a standing position, hands on hips. Step forward with the right foot, bending on one knee and dipping, with your left leg outstretched behind you. Step back to the starting position. Step forward with the right foot, repeating dipping and outstretching motions. For the thighs (quads and hamstrings).

8. **Three-way leg lift.** Stand near a wall or piece of furniture for support. While standing on your left leg with the knee straight but not locked, slowly raise the right leg, with the toe pointed, straight up in front of you, six to twelve inches. Hold for two seconds.

In a smooth motion, return your leg to the side and slowly bring your extended leg out to the right, lifting six to twelve inches from the ground, toes pointed. Hold for two seconds.

Again in a smooth motion, return to the beginning position and slowly extend the leg out behind you, lifting six to twelve inches off the ground, toes pointed. Hold for two seconds. Return your leg to the beginning position.

Repeat with the left leg. You should gradually build to do this exercise without resting between position changes. For added resistance, use light ankle weights. For hips/buttocks and thighs (gluteals, quads, and hamstrings).

9. **Heel lifts.** Stand on one step, balancing on the balls of your feet, near a wall or railing. Slowly rise up onto your toes, hold for two seconds, then return to a balanced position. Now let your heels drop off the step, hold for one second, and return to a balanced position. This can also be done one foot at a time, or with ankle weights. For calves, ankles, and feet.

10. **Classic curl.** Stand with legs about shoulder width apart. Grasp a dumbbell with each hand, arms extended at the side, palms facing in. Bending at the elbows, curl the weight in toward your body, up to about shoulder height. Your palms should be facing you as you lift the weights. You can do both arms at the same time, or alternate.

Remember to breathe smoothly as you lift. For front of the arms (biceps).

11. **Triceps teaser.** Standing with legs about shoulder-width apart, grasp the end of *one* dumbbell with *both* hands and place your arms above your head. Your elbows should be bent, your hands grasping the weight behind your head. Slowly extend both arms over your head, hold for two seconds, and return to the starting position. For back of the arms.

Safety Tips For Strength Training

■ **Always warm up before you train, and cool down after your session.** It pays off in a safer, more comfortable workout.

■ **Pay attention to previous injuries.** If you have a knee problem, for example, get advice about how to compensate for that injury from the fitness director at your club, from a physician who specializes in sports medicine, or from a physical therapist.

■ **Stop training if you feel pain.** That's a signal you're overdoing it.

■ **Start with larger muscle groups and work down to the smaller ones.** When training the larger muscle groups, do so in the following order: abdominals to work the back and stomach muscles; the legs; then the chest and back.

To train the smaller muscle groups, start with the shoulders, work the biceps (front of upper arm), then finish with the triceps (back of upper arm). Strength-training circuits at most clubs are arranged in this order.

■ **Use proper posture.** When standing, make sure your feet are shoulder-width apart. Don't lock your elbows or knees; it puts undue strain on them. Keep weight well balanced, without leaning to one side or the other. Keep head and neck straight, making sure not to twist either. Keep your back flat and straight, making sure not to arch it or twist during any strength-training activity.

■ **Use only the proper muscles.** Avoid using muscles other than the one you're exercising. For example, if you're using the leg-curl machine, you should feel a pulling in the back of your thighs. If you feel it in your back as well, you're probably arching your back and using the wrong muscles.

■ **Lift with a smooth, dynamic motion.** You know your muscle is too tired when you can no longer lift smoothly.

■ **Breathe properly.** Exhale when lifting, inhale when returning. Whatever you do, don't hold your breath during any part of your training. Holding your breath tends to raise your blood pressure, which may result in dizziness or even a blackout.

■ **Take special care when using the back-extension machine (Roman chair).** Start with little or no weight, and add weight very gradually. While this machine can be very useful in building back muscles, using too much weight too soon can cause injury.

■ **Use common sense.** Pads and strapping are provided for your safety. Use them when provided. Follow diagrams on machines for proper use. If a strength-training machine is too big for you, find an alternative or get the proper instruction on how to use the appropriate free weights instead. If you use a machine that's too big, you'll be using all the wrong muscles, which can cause injury.

(Taken from *The Exercise Exchange Program* by Dr. James M. Rippe, New York: Simon & Schuster, 1992)

THE POLAR HEART RATE MONITOR

Whether your exercise of choice is running indoors or outdoors, step aerobics at home or at the club, walking on a treadmill or outside or bicycling on a stationary cycle use your Polar Heart Rate Monitor. With a simple glimpse at your wrist, you will know whether you are in your Weight Management Zone or, later in your program, the Aerobic Training Zone. You will know, without missing a beat, whether your exercise is effectively burning calories — and keeping you fit.

The quickest way to become familiar with your Polar Heart Rate Monitor is to read the easy-to-understand Instruction Manual that comes with the product. It will help you to use your Polar Heart Rate Monitor correctly from the start.

Here are a couple of important things you should know about the Polar Heart Rate Monitor that makes it the most accurate fitness monitor in the world — and the reasons why it is the choice of health and fitness professionals everywhere.

THE CHEST TRANSMITTER: THE HEART OF THE PRODUCT

When you strap on the lightweight, comfortable heart rate transmitter, you are putting on the only wireless monitor that has been proven in clinical testing facilities to be as accurate as a doctor's electrocardiogram in monitoring the beats of the heart. This is accomplished by sensitive electrodes encased in the chestbelt transmitter that monitor your heart rate changes constantly. The accuracy of the Polar Heart Rate Monitor wireless transmitter makes it sensitive to your body's constant change in heart rate as you exercise. This high level of accuracy enables you to take the "guesswork" out of exercise and to know when your body is being exercised at effective and safe levels of intensity.

Many studies have proven that Polar Heart Rate Monitors are the key to effective weight loss and fitness because of their accuracy in showing when a person's heart is being exercised in the proper target heart rate zone. So take heart and monitor your heart — and use the Polar Heart Rate Monitor to keep yourself trim, fit, and healthy.

THE WRIST MONITOR: THE WINDOW TO YOUR HEART

The Polar wristwatch receiver works by picking up the changes in your heart rate as it is being monitored and transmitted by the wireless chestbelt transmitter. The wristwatch receiver displays the constant changes in your heart rate as you exercise — so you always know when you are in your effective target heart rate zone. Most Polar Heart Rate Monitors also function as an accurate watch showing time of day — so you can track your exercise time at the same time you monitor your target heart rate zone.

See Appendix A (page 143) for the range of Polar Heart Rate Monitors and their features. Since Polar is constantly adding to its line of products, have your local Polar retailer explain which model is right for you. Call 1-800-227-1314 for the Polar retailer nearest you.

• • • • • • • •

That's all there is to it. You now have your individual Polar Exercise Program, complete with a 20-week regime in the exercise of your choice, strength training suggestions, stretches, warm-ups and cool-downs — and some basic instructions on how to use your Polar Heart Rate Monitor to the max. But getting fit is only half the story. Your exercise program must be used in conjunction with your food program — coming up next. . . .

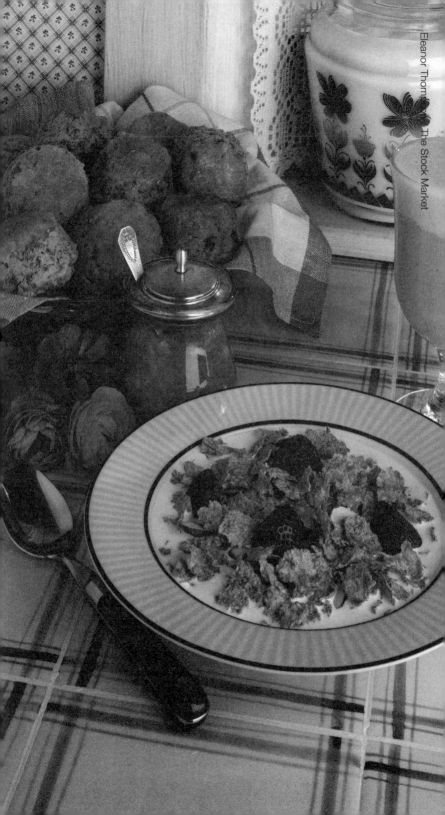

Your Three-Step Polar Nutrition Program

"The best part of the program is the food.
I'm never hungry.
I don't feel deprived. This isn't a diet!"

—A 53-year-old small business owner who's been on the Polar Program
for two months

The food you eat is as important as the amount of exercise
you get. In the Polar equation, fat free and fit forever means eating a
nutritious, healthy diet — that you can live with your whole life long.

The Polar Nutrition Program has three "Eat Smart" steps that
lead to weight management success:

Eat Smart Step # 1:
DETERMINING YOUR INDIVIDUAL MEAL PLAN

Losing weight is easy — if you recognize the truism that slow and steady wins the race. The goal is to achieve the kind of lifelong, low-fat eating principles which, together with regular exercise, assures permanent weight management. The diet plan in the Polar Fat Free and Fit Forever Program is based on a loss of one to two pounds of fat a week. This may not sound like much, especially when you're impatient to lose weight fast, but one pound a week equals 52 pounds a year! And, because there's no deprivation involved, no impossible absolutes or sacrifice, you'll stay with it, as opposed to all those countless diets where you end up gaining back all your weight — over and over again!

The people who participated in our Polar study at the Exercise Physiology and Nutrition Laboratory found the diet easy to use and easy to live with. We think you will, too. It's based on three different meal plans: 1,200, 1,500, and 1,800 calories a day. How do you know which is the right meal plan for you?

The process is really quite simple:

1. **Add a zero to your current weight.** This will tell you the number of calories you need to maintain it. For example, if you weighed 150 pounds, you'd need to take in 1,500 calories a day to maintain it.

2. **Determine how many calories you need to lose a pound a week.** As we discussed in Chapter One, you need to burn 500 calories a day (or 3,500 calories a week) to lose one

pound. Using the same example above, the 150 pound individual would need a diet of 1,000 calories to lose that pound a week:

$$1,500 - 500 = 1,000 \text{ calories a day}$$

3. **Add 200 calories for exercise.** The same 150 pound person above has started exercise. If he is using his Polar Heart Rate Monitor and staying in his Weight Management Zone, he is burning 200 extra calories a day — *which should be added to the meal plan equation.*

$$200 \text{ "exercise" calories} + 1,000 \text{ "diet" calories} = 1,200$$

4. **Pick your meal plan.** The man above would start on the 1,200 calorie a day plan, enough to lose one or two pounds a week without deprivation.

That's all there is to it. But what if you fall somewhere in between our three meal plans? No problem. You just have to make a few adjustments. Let's try an example using the above steps:

If, say, you weigh 140 pounds, you would need 1,400 calories a day to maintain it. Subtract the prerequisite 500 calories a day to lose one pound a week (1,400 – 500 = 900.) Add your 200 "exercise" calories and you have a total of 1,100 calories per day.

$$200 \text{ "exercise" calories} + 900 \text{ "diet" calories} = 1,100$$

Your best choice here is to go with the 1,200 calorie plan. Anything less could be harmful to your health. Sticking with 1,200 ensures good health — plus you'll still lose weight. And, as the weeks go by, you'll be adding more exercise to your Polar regimen — and you'll burn even more calories.

On the other hand, perhaps you weigh 220 pounds and want to go on the Polar Program. You'd need 2,200 calories a day to maintain your weight. Subtract the 500 calories you need to burn to lose a pound a week (2,200 − 500 = 1,700) and you're left with 1,700. Add the 200 "exercise" calories and you have a total of 1,900 calories a day.

200 "exercise" calories + 1,700 "diet" calories = 1,900

Your best choice here is to go with the 1,800 Calorie Meal Plan. More than that and you'll be consuming too much fat.

As you choose your meal plan, remember that flexibility is key. Nothing is etched in stone. If your equation tells you to start with the 1,800 Calorie Meal Plan, but you don't lose weight within a month, drop down to the 1,500 Calorie Meal Plan. Similarly, if you're on, say, the 1,200 Calorie Meal Plan, but you're losing more than two pounds a week, you should move up to the 1,500 Calorie Meal Plan for good health and safe weight loss management.

Eat Smart Step # 2:
LEARNING TO USE YOUR FOOD EXCHANGES

Don't be alarmed at the numbers. Even though your meal plans are based on calories, we've done the work for you. As you read in Chapter Two, we use a system of food exchanges that have been developed by the American Dietetic Association and the American Diabetes Association. Each meal plan, 1,200, 1,500, and 1,800, have different "exchange" requirements within the six food categories (Protein/Meat, Starch/Bread,

Vegetable, Fruit, Fat, and Milk). These detailed Food Exchange Lists follow on the next few pages. In addition to the exchanges each Meal Plan requires, each Plan also comes with "Open Calories." These are extra calories you can consume every day. You can pick your "Open Calories" from the food exchange lists that end this chapter or from any calorie counter booklet. Try to keep your Fat "Open Calories" to a minimum for faster weight loss and better health.

Here are the exchanges for each meal plan:

1,200 Calories a Day Meal Plan Exchanges

4 Starch/Bread	3 Fruit
4 Protein/Meat	2 Milk
3 Vegetable	3 Fat

80 Open Calories

1,500 Calories a Day Meal Plan Exchanges

5 Starch/Bread	4 Fruit
5 Protein/Meat	2 Milk
3 Vegetable	3 Fat

200 Open Calories

1,800 Calories a Day Meal Plan Exchanges

6 Starch/Bread	4 Fruit
6 Protein/Meat	2 Milk
4 Vegetable	4 Fat

300 Open Calories

We've included a blank food diary in the Appendix that you can copy and use to keep track of your exchanges every day. You'll also find in the Appendix a pocket-sized "recap" of the exchanges required for each of the three Meal Plans.

Eat Smart Step # 3: MEASURING FOOD

Remember your 3Ms for staying on track. One of them was **Measuring.** The exchanges you use every day are based on serving size. In order to eat the correct portions you'll need to measure your food — at least initially. Use measuring cups and spoons; a weight control scale will also help. The Food Lists that follow also contain some tips on portion size and scale. It may seem cumbersome at first to weigh and measure, but in the long run it insures that you are following the program correctly. Too little food and you might not be getting the nutrients you need. Too much and you won't lose the weight you want. And, in time, the need to measure will decrease. You'll be able to estimate portion size more accurately — at home, in restaurants, or wherever you dine.

• • • • • • • •

This is it. The Polar Fat Free and Fit Forever Program. You now have everything you need to get on track. But, since everybody appreciates a helping hand, turn to the next chapter for some hints and tips to make your Polar Program the experience of a lifetime!

Food Exchange Lists

The foods listed within each category have approximately the same amount of protein, fat, carbohydrate, and calories per serving. *Every food is listed with a serving size that equals one exchange.*

STARCH/BREAD LIST

Each item in this list contains approximately 15 grams of carbohydrates, 3 grams of protein, a trace of fat, and 80 calories. Whole-grain products average about 2 grams of fiber per exchange. Some foods are higher in fiber. Those foods that contain 3 or more grams of fiber per exchange are footnoted.

You can choose your starch exchanges from any of the items on this list. If you want to eat a starch food that is not on this list, the general rule is that:

- ½ cup of cereal, grain, or pasta is one exchange
- 1 ounce of a bread product is one exchange

CEREALS/GRAINS/PASTA

Bran cereals,* concentrated (such as Bran Buds, All Bran)	⅓ cup
Bran cereals,* flaked	½ cup
Bulgur (cooked)	½ cup
Cooked cereals	½ cup
Cornmeal (dry)	2½ tbsp
Grape-Nuts	3 tbsp.
Grits (cooked)	½ cup
Other ready-to-eat unsweetened cereals	¾ cup
Pasta (cooked)	½ cup
Puffed cereal	1½ cups
Rice, white or brown (cooked)	⅓ cup
Shredded wheat	½ cup
Wheat germ*	3 tbsp.

*3 g. or more of fiber per exchange.

* The Exchange Lists are the bases of a meal planning system designed by a committee of the American Diabetes Association and the American Dietetic Association. While designed primarily for people with diabetes and others who must follow special diets, the exchange lists are based on principles of good nutrition that apply to everyone. Copyright © 1989 by the American Diabetes Association, and the American Dietetic Association.

(The lists on the next 17 pages are taken from *The Rockport Walking Program* by Dr. James M. Rippe, Ann Ward, Ph.D., with Karla Dougherty, New York: Fireside Press, 1989, and *The Exercise Exchange Program* by Dr. James M. Rippe, New York: Simon & Schuster, 1992)

DRIED BEANS/PEAS/LENTILS

Beans* and peas* (cooked),	⅓ cup
such as kidney, white, split, black-eyed	
Lentils* (cooked)	⅓ cup
Baked beans*	¼ cup

*3 g. or more of fiber per exchange.

STARCHY VEGETABLES

Corn*	½ cup
Corn on cob,* 6 in. long	1
Lima beans*	½ cup
Peas, green* (canned or frozen)	½ cup
Plantain*	½ cup
Potato, baked	1 small (3 oz.)
Potato, mashed	½ cup
Squash, winter* (acorn, butternut)	¾ cup
Yam, sweet potato, plain	⅓ cup

*3 g. or more of fiber per exchange.

BREAD

Bagel	½ (1 oz.)
Breadsticks, crisp, 4 in. long × ½ in.	2 (⅔ oz.)
Croutons, low-fat	1 cup
English muffin	½
Frankfurter or hamburger bun	½ (1 oz.)
Pita, 6 in. across	½
Plain roll, small	1 (1 oz.)
Raisin, unfrosted	1 slice (1 oz.)
Rye, pumpernickel	1 slice (1 oz.)
Tortilla, 6 in. across	1
White (including French, Italian)	1 slice (1 oz.)
Whole wheat	1 slice (1 oz.)

CRACKERS/SNACKS

Animal crackers	8
Graham crackers, 2½ in. square	3
Matzoh	¾ oz.
Melba toast	5 slices
Oyster crackers	24
Popcorn (popped, no fat added)	3 cups
Pretzels	¾ oz.
Ry-Krisp,* 2 in. × 3½ in.	4
Saltine-type crackers	6
Whole-wheat crackers,*	2–4 slices (¾ oz.)
no fat added (crisp breads, such as	
Finn, Kavli, Wasa)	

*3 g. or more of fiber per exchange.

STARCH FOODS PREPARED WITH FAT

COUNT AS 1 STARCH/BREAD EXCHANGE, PLUS 1 FAT EXCHANGE

Biscuit, 2½ in. across	1
Chow mein noodles	½ cup
Corn bread, 2-in. cube	1 (2 oz.)
Cracker, round butter type	6
French-fried potatoes, 2 in. to 3½ in. long	10 (1½ oz.)
Muffin, plain, small	1
Pancake, 4 in. across	2
Stuffing, bread (prepared)	¼ cup
Taco shell, 6 in. across	2
Waffle, 4½ in. square	1
Whole-wheat crackers,*	4–6 (1 oz.)
fat added (such as Triscuit)	

*3 g. or more of fiber per exchange.

MEAT LIST

Each serving of meat and substitutes in this list contains about 7 grams of protein. The amount of fat and number of calories varies, depending on what kind of meat or substitute you choose. The list is divided into three parts based on the amount of fat and calories: lean meat, medium-fat meat, and high-fat meat. One ounce (one meat exchange) of each of these includes:

	Carbohydrate (Grams)	Protein (Grams)	Fat (Grams)	Calories
Lean	0	7	3	55
Medium-fat	0	7	5	75
High-fat	0	7	8	100

You are encouraged to use lean meat, poultry, and fish in your meal plan. This will help decrease your fat intake, which may help decrease your risk of heart disease. The items from the high-fat group are high in saturated fat, cholesterol, and calories. Meat and substitutes do not contribute any fiber to your meal plan.

Meats and meat substitutes that have 400 milligrams or more of sodium per exchange are footnoted.

Meats and meat substitutes that have 400 milligrams or more of sodium if two or more exchanges are eaten are footnoted.

TIPS

- Bake, roast, broil, grill, or boil these foods rather than frying them with added fat.
- Use a nonstick pan spray or a nonstick pan to brown or fry these foods.
- Trim off visible fat before and after cooking.
- Do not add flour, bread crumbs, coating mixes, or fat to these foods when preparing them.
- Weigh meat after removing bones and fat, and after cooking. Three ounces of cooked meat is about equal to 4 ounces of raw meat. Some examples of meat portions are:

  2 ounces meat (2 meat exchanges) =
    1 small chicken leg or thigh
    ½ cup cottage cheese or tuna
  3 ounces meat (3 meat exchanges) =
    1 medium pork chop
    1 small hamburger
    ½ whole chicken breast
    1 unbreaded fish fillet
    cooked meat, about the size of a deck of cards

- Restaurants usually serve prime cuts of meat, which are high in fat and calories.

LEAN MEAT AND SUBSTITUTES

One exchange is equal to any one of the following items:

Beef	USDA Select or Choice grades of lean beef, such as round, sirloin, and flank steak; tenderloin; and chipped beef*	1 oz.
Pork	Lean pork, such as fresh ham; canned, cured, or boiled ham,* Canadian bacon,* tenderloin	1 oz.
Veal	All cuts are lean except for veal cutlets (ground or cubed); examples of lean veal are chops and roasts	1 oz.
Poultry	Chicken, turkey, Cornish hen (without skin)	1 oz.
Fish	All fresh and frozen fish	1 oz.
	Crab, lobster, scallops, shrimp, clams (fresh or canned in water)	2 oz.
	Oysters	6 medium
	Tuna† (canned in water)	¼ cup
	Herring† (uncreamed or smoked)	1 oz.
	Sardines (canned)	2 medium
Wild game	Venison, rabbit, squirrel	1 oz.
	Pheasant, duck, goose (without skin)	1 oz.
Cheese	Any cottage cheese†	¼ cup
	Grated Parmesan	2 tbsp.
	Diet cheeses* (with less than 55 calories per ounce)	1 oz.
Other	95 percent fat-free luncheon meat*	1 oz.
	Egg whites	3 whites
	Egg substitutes with less than 55 calories per cup	¼ cup

*400 mg. or more of sodium per exchange.
†400 mg. or more of sodium if two or more exchanges are eaten.

MEDIUM-FAT MEAT AND SUBSTITUTES

One exchange is equal to any one of the following items:

Beef	Most beef products fall into this category, such as all ground beef, roast (rib, chuck, rump), steak (cubed, porterhouse, T-bone), and meat loaf	1 oz.
Pork	Most pork products fall into this category, such as chops, loin roast, Boston butt and cutlets	1 oz.
Lamb	Most lamb products fall into this category, such as chops, leg, and roast	1 oz.
Veal	Cutlet (ground or cubed, unbreaded)	1 oz.
Poultry	Chicken (with skin), domestic duck or goose (well drained of fat), ground turkey	1 oz.
Fish	Tuna* (canned in oil and drained)	¼ cup
	Salmon* (canned)	¼ cup
Cheese	Skim or part-skim milk cheeses, such as	
	Ricotta	¼ cup
	Mozzarella	1 oz.
	Diet cheeses (with 56–80 calories per ounce)	1 oz.
Other	86 percent fat-free luncheon meat*	1 oz.
	Egg (high in cholesterol, limit to 3 per week)	1
	Egg substitutes with 56–80 calories per ¼ cup	¼ cup
	Tofu (2½ in. × 2¾ in. × 1 in.)	4 oz.
	Liver, heart, kidney, sweetbreads (high in cholesterol)	1 oz.

*400 mg. or more of sodium if two or more exchanges are eaten.
†400 mg. or more of sodium per exchange.

HIGH-FAT MEAT AND SUBSTITUTES

Remember, these items are high in saturated fat, cholesterol, and calories. One exchange is equal to any one of the following items.

Beef	Most USDA prime cuts of beef, such as ribs, corned beef*	1 oz.
Pork	Spareribs, ground pork, pork sausage† (patty or link)	1 oz.
Lamb	Patties (ground lamb)	1 oz.
Fish:	Any fried fish product	1 oz.
Cheese	All regular cheeses, such as American,† Blue,† Cheddar,† Monterey Jack,† Swiss	1 oz.
Other	Luncheon meat such as bologna, salami, pimento loaf†	1 oz.
	Sausage,† such as Polish, Italian smoked	1 oz.
	Knockwurst†	1 oz.
	Bratwurst*	1 oz.
	Frankfurter† (turkey or chicken)	1 frank (10/lb.)
	Peanut butter (contains unsaturated fat)	1 tbsp.

Count as one high-fat meat plus one fat exchange

	Frankfurter† (beef, pork, or combination)	1 frank (10/lb.)

*400 mg. or more of sodium if two or more exchanges are eaten.
†400 mg. or more of sodium per exchange.

VEGETABLE LIST

Each vegetable serving in this list contains about 5 grams of carbohydrates, 2 grams of protein, and 25 calories. Vegetables contain 2 to 3 grams of dietary fiber. Vegetables that contain 400 milligrams or more of sodium per exchange are footnoted.

Vegetables are good sources of vitamins and minerals. Fresh and frozen vegetables have more vitamins and less added salt. Rinsing canned vegetables will remove much of the salt.

Unless otherwise noted, the serving size for vegetables (one vegetable exchange) is:

- ½ cup of cooked vegetables or vegetable juice
- 1 cup of raw vegetables

Starchy vegetables such as corn, peas, and potatoes are in the starch/bread list.

Artichoke (½ medium)	Mushrooms, cooked
Asparagus	Okra
Beans (green, wax, Italian)	Onions
Bean sprouts	Pea pods
Beets	Peppers (green)
Broccoli	Rutabaga
Brussels sprouts	Sauerkraut*
Cabbage, cooked	Spinach, cooked
Carrots	Summer squash (crookneck)
Cauliflower	Tomato (one large)
Eggplant	Tomato/vegetable juice*
Greens (collard, mustard, turnip)	Turnips
Kohlrabi	Water chestnuts
Leeks	Zucchini, cooked

*400 mg. or more of sodium per exchange.

FRUIT LIST

Each item in this list contains about 15 grams of carbohydrates and 60 calories. Fresh, frozen, and dried fruits have about 2 grams of fiber per exchange. Fruits that have 3 or more grams of fiber per exchange are footnoted.

The carbohydrate and calorie contents for a fruit exchange are based on the usual serving of the most commonly eaten fruits. Use fresh fruits or fruits frozen or canned without sugar added. Whole fruit is more filling than fruit juice and may be a better choice for those who are trying to lose weight. Unless otherwise noted, the serving size for one fruit exchange is:

- ½ cup of fresh fruit or fruit juice
- ¼ cup of dried fruit

FRESH, FROZEN, AND UNSWEETENED CANNED FRUIT

Apple (raw, 2 in. across)	1 apple
Applesauce (unsweetened)	½ cup
Apricots (medium, raw)	4 apricots
Apricots (canned)	½ cup, or 4 halves
Banana (9 in. long)	½ banana
Blackberries* (raw)	¾ cup
Blueberries* (raw)	¾ cup
Cantaloupe (5 in. across)	⅓ melon
(cubes)	1 cup
Cherries (large, raw)	12 cherries
Cherries (canned)	½ cup
Figs (raw, 2 in. across)	2 figs
Fruit cocktail (canned)	½ cup
Grapefruit (medium)	½ grapefruit
Grapefruit (segments)	¾ cup
Grapes (small)	15 grapes
Honeydew melon (medium)	⅛ melon
(cubes)	1 cup
Kiwi (large)	1 kiwi
Mandarin oranges	¾ cup
Mango (small)	½ mango
Nectarine* (2½ in. across)	1 nectarine
Orange (2½ in. across)	1 orange
Papaya	1 cup
Peach (2¾ in. across)	1 peach, or ¾ cup
Peaches (canned)	½ cup, or 2 halves
Pear	½ large, or 1 small
Pears (canned)	½ cup, or 2 halves
Persimmon (medium, native)	2 persimmons
Pineapple (raw)	¾ cup
Pineapple (canned)	⅓ cup
Plum (raw, 2 in. across)	2 plums
Pomegranate*	½ pomegranate
Raspberries* (raw)	1 cup
Strawberries* (raw, whole)	1¼ cup
Tangerine* (2½ in. across)	2 tangerines
Watermelon (cubes)	1¼ cup

3 g. or more of fiber per exchange.

DRIED FRUIT

Apples*	4 rings
Apricots*	7 halves
Dates	2½ medium
Figs*	1½
Prunes*	3 medium
Raisins	2 tbsp.

3 g. or more of fiber per exchange.

FRUIT JUICE

Apple juice/cider	½ cup
Cranberry juice cocktail	⅓ cup
Grapefruit juice	½ cup
Grape juice	⅓ cup
Orange juice	½ cup
Pineapple juice	½ cup
Prune juice	⅓ cup

MILK LIST

Each serving of milk or milk products in this list contains about 12 grams of carbohydrates and 8 grams of protein. The amount of fat in milk is measured in percent of butterfat. The calories vary, depending on what kind of milk you choose. The list is divided into three parts, based on the amount of fat and calories: skim/very low-fat milk, low-fat milk, and whole milk. One serving (one milk exchange) of each of these includes:

	Carbohydrate (grams)	Protein (Grams)	Fat (Grams)	Calories
Skim/very low-fat	12	8	trace	90
Low-fat	12	8	5	120
Whole	12	8	8	150

Milk is the body's main source of calcium, the mineral needed for growth and repair of bones. Yogurt is also a good source of calcium. Yogurt and many dry or powdered milk products have different amounts of fat. If you have questions about a particular item, read the label to find out the fat and calorie content.

Milk is good to drink, but it can also be added to cereal and to other foods.

SKIM AND VERY LOW-FAT MILK

Skim milk	1 cup
½ percent milk	1 cup
1 percent milk	1 cup
Low-fat buttermilk	1 cup
Evaporated skim milk	½ cup
Dry nonfat milk	⅓ cup
Plain nonfat yogurt	8 oz.

LOW-FAT MILK

2 percent milk	1 cup fluid
Plain low-fat yogurt (with added nonfat milk solids)	8 oz.

WHOLE MILK

The whole milk group has much more fat per serving than the skim and lowfat groups. Whole milk has more than 3¼ percent butterfat. Try to limit your choices from the whole milk group as much as possible.

Whole milk	1 cup
Evaporated whole milk	½ cup
Whole plain yogurt	8 oz.

FAT LIST

Each serving in this list contains about 5 grams of fat and 45 calories.

The foods in this list contain mostly fat, although some items may also contain a small amount of protein. All fats are high in calories and should be carefully measured. Everyone should modify fat intake by eating unsaturated fats instead of saturated fats.

UNSATURATED FATS

Avocado	⅛ medium
Margarine	1 tsp.
Margarine* diet	1 tbsp.
Mayonnaise	1 tsp.
Mayonnaise* reduced-calorie	1 tbsp.
Nuts and seeds:	
Almonds, dry roasted	6 whole
Cashews, dry roasted	1 tbsp.
Pecans	2 whole
Peanuts	20 small or 10 large
Walnuts	2 whole
Other nuts	1 tbsp.
Seeds, pine nuts, sunflower (without shells)	1 tbsp.
Pumpkin seeds	2 tsp.
Oil (corn, cottonseed, safflower, soybean, sunflower, olive, peanut)	1 tsp.
Olives*	10 small or 5 large
Salad dressing, mayonnaise-type	2 tsp.
Salad dressing, mayonnaise-type, reduced-calorie	1 tbsp.
Salad dressing* (oil varieties)	1 tbsp.
Salad dressing,† reduced-calorie	2 tbsp.

*400 mg. or more of sodium if two or more exchanges are eaten.
†400 mg. or more of sodium per exchange.

SATURATED FATS

Butter	1 tsp.
Bacon*	1 slice
Chitterlings	½ ounce
Coconut, shredded	2 tbsp.
Coffee whitener, liquid	2 tbsp.
Coffee whitener, powder	4 tsp.
Cream (light, coffee, table)	2 tbsp.
Cream, sour	2 tbsp.
Cream (heavy, whipping)	1 tbsp.
Cream cheese	1 tbsp.
Salt pork*	¼ ounce

*400 mg. or more of sodium if two or more exchanges are eaten.

FREE FOODS

A free food is any food or drink that contains less than 20 calories per serving. You can eat as much as you want of those items that have no serving size specified. You may eat two or three servings per day of those items that have a specific serving size. Be sure to spread them out through the day.

DRINKS

Bouillon, or broth without fat*
Bouillon, low-sodium
Carbonated drinks, sugar-free
Carbonated water
Club soda

Cocoa powder, unsweetened (1 tbsp.)
Coffee/tea
Drink mixes, sugar-free
Tonic water, sugar-free

*400 mg. or more of sodium per exchange.

NONSTICK PAN SPRAY

FRUIT

Cranberries, unsweetened (½ cup)   Rhubarb, unsweetened (½ cup)

VEGETABLES (raw, 1 cup)

Cabbage
Celery
Chinese cabbage*
Cucumber
Green onion

Hot peppers
Mushrooms
Radishes
Zucchini*

*3 g. or more of fiber per exchange.

SALAD GREENS

Endive
Escarole
Lettuce

Romaine
Spinach

SWEET SUBSTITUTES

Candy, hard, sugar-free
Gelatin, sugar-free
Gum, sugar-free
Jam/jelly, sugar-free
(less than 20 cal./2 tsp.)

Pancake syrup, sugar-free (1–2 tbsp.)
Sugar substitutes (saccharin, aspartame)
Whipped topping (2 tbsp.)

CONDIMENTS

Ketchup (1 tbsp.)
Horseradish
Mustard
Pickles,* dill, unsweetened

Salad dressing,† low-calorie (2 tbsp.)
Taco sauce (1 tbsp.)
Vinegar

*400 mg. or more of sodium per exchange.
†The nutritionists who developed the diet for *The Rockport Walking Program* suggest that only those salad dressings with 10 calories or less per tablespoon be considered "free foods."

Seasonings (see the following material) can be very helpful in making food taste better. Be careful of how much sodium you use. Read the label, and choose those seasonings that do not contain sodium or salt.

SEASONINGS

Basil (fresh)
Celery seeds
Chili powder
Chives
Cinnamon
Curry
Dill
Flavoring extracts (vanilla, almond, walnut, peppermint, butter, lemon, etc.)
Garlic
Garlic powder
Herbs
Hot pepper sauce
Lemon
Lemon juice

Lemon pepper
Lime
Lime juice
Mint
Onion powder
Oregano
Paprika
Pepper
Pimento
Spices
Soy sauce*
Soy sauce,* low-sodium ("lite")
Wine, used in cooking (¼ cup)
Worcestershire sauce

*400 mg. or more of sodium per exchange.

COMBINATION FOODS

Much of the food we eat is mixed in various combinations. These combination foods do not fit into only one exchange list. It can be quite hard to tell what is in a certain casserole dish or baked food item. This is a list of average values for some typical combination foods. This list will help you fit these foods into your meal plans.

Food	Amount	Exchanges
Casseroles, homemade	1 cup (8 oz.)	2 starch, 2 medium-fat meat, 1 fat
Cheese pizza,* thin crust	¼ of 15 oz., or ¼ of 10"	2 starch, 1 medium-fat meat, 1 fat
Chili with beans*† (commercial)	1 cup (8 oz.)	2 starch, 2 medium-fat meat, 2 fat
Chow mein* (without noodles or rice)	2 cups (16 oz.)	1 starch, 2 vegetable, 2 lean meat
Macaroni and cheese*	1 cup (8 oz.)	2 starch, 1 medium-fat meat, 2 fat
Soup		
Bean*†	1 cup (8 oz.)	1 starch, 1 vegetable, 1 lean meat
Chunky, all varieties*	10¾ oz. can	1 starch, 1 vegetable, 1 medium-fat meat
Cream* (made with water)	1 cup (8 oz.)	1 starch, 1 fat
Vegetable* or broth-type*	1 cup (8 oz.)	1 starch
Spaghetti and meatballs* (canned)	1 cup (8 oz.)	2 starch, 1 medium-fat meat, 1 fat
If beans are used as a meat substitute		
Dried beans,† peas,† lentils	1 cup (cooked)	2 starch, 1 lean meat

*400 mg. or more of sodium per exchange.
†3 g. or more of fiber per exchange.

ADDITIONAL EXCHANGE LIST*

Starch/Bread List

Bread, low-calorie (40 calories per slice)	2 slices
Bread crumbs, dried	3 tbsp.
Rice cakes	2
Zwieback cookies	2
Arrowroot cookies	4
Vanilla wafers	5
Gingersnaps	3
Flour	3 tbsp.
Cornstarch	3 tbsp.
Lowfat cookies	¾ oz.

Vegetable List

Mixed vegetables (frozen)	⅓ cup
Peas and carrots (frozen)	⅓ cup

Fat List

Tartar sauce	2 tsp.

Milk List

Sugar-free hot cocoa (40 calories)	2 packets
Sugar-free pudding made with skim milk	½ cup
Sugar-free shake mix (70 calories)	1 packet
Fruited yogurt, nonfat, any flavor	½ cup
Frozen yogurt, low-fat, any flavor	½ cup
Frozen yogurt bar, low-fat	1 bar
Fudge bar, Fudgsicle, etc.†	1 bar
Ice milk (no more than 110 calories per serving)	½ cup

Additional Combination Foods

Refried beans	⅓ cup	1 starch, 1 fat
Fruited yogurt, Any flavor, low-fat	1 cup	1 milk, 2 fruit, ½ fat
Granola	¼ cup	1 starch, 1 fat
Granola bar	1 small	1 starch, 1 fat
Snack chips	1 ounce	1 starch, 2 fat
Microwave popcorn	3½ cups (or ⅓ of a 10-cup bag)	1 starch, 1 fat

*Adapted with permission from *The Rockport Walking Program* (New York: Prentice Hall, 1989).
†There are many low-calorie frozen desserts on the market today. Many of them are made with low-fat milk and have less than 100 calories. These may be included in the diet and counted as one milk exchange.

ADDITIONAL FREE FOODS*

Seasonings
Flavored crystals (Butter Buds, Molly McButter, etc.)
Crystal Light Bars (14 calories/bar)
Tabasco
Salsa
Teriyaki
Salt
Celery salt
Garlic salt
Onion salt
All spices and herbs
Ginger, fresh or powder
Tenderizers
No-oil salad dressing

Alcohol

We stress moderation here, not only because of the obvious physical and psychological dangers of too much alcohol but also because alcohol provides calories and not much else in the way of nutrition. And with seven calories per gram, alcohol nearly matches fat's nine calories per gram.

Type	Amount	Exchange
Table wine	4 oz.	2 fats
Beer	12 oz.	1 starch, 2 fats
Beer, light	12 oz.	2 fats
Whiskey, gin, vodka, Scotch, etc.	1.5 oz. (1 shot)	2 fats

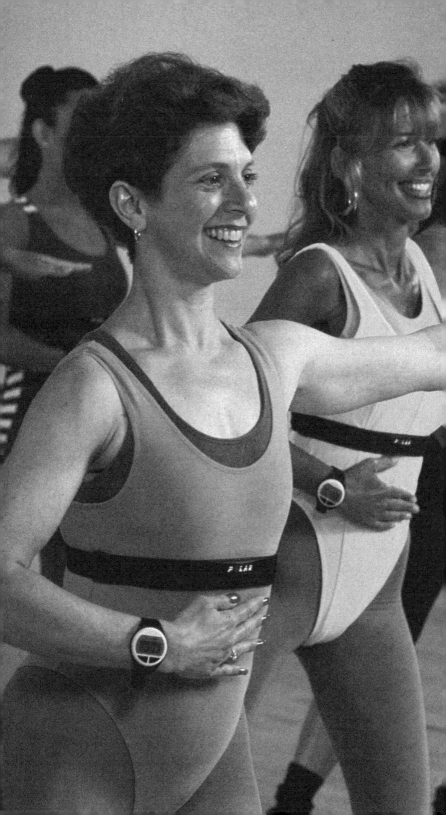

"The best part of this Program?

The

The long-term outlook.

Polar

I know what works for the long run.

Program:

Even better,

Staying

I know I can do it for nothing less than the rest of my life."

Started

—A 39-year-old marketing manager who's been on
the Polar Fat Free and Fit Forever Program for over one year

Ask anyone who's ever been on a weight loss program
and they'll tell you: The hardest part of losing weight isn't the
day-to-day dieting. It's keeping it off. The Polar Fat Free and Fit
Forever Program recognizes this difficulty — and has some
suggestions to help keep your long-term motivation strong and, at

the same time, substitute good habits for the bad ones that have kept you unhealthy for too long. It's not magic. It's a matter of incorporating healthy eating and exercise habits into your day-to-day routine — until they become a part of your daily life, as necessary and as "rote" as picking up food for dinner or washing your hair.

That's why I like to think of exercise as **increased** activity. There's more to life — and increased activity — than the 20-week exercise options I've outlined for you within these pages. Believe it or not, mowing the lawn can burn calories. So can sweeping or stacking firewood. Even washing and drying clothes have their place in aerobic activity. That's why I've helped design exercise exchanges for the Polar Fat Free and Fit Forever Program. On the following pages, you will find daily activities and the minutes you need to perform them to burn 100 calories. Use these activities on the days you just don't feel like getting on the Lifecycle or walking around the block. Double the minutes and you still have the 200 "exercise" calories you need every day in your weight loss equation. In short, these charts can help insure that increased activity becomes integrated into your lifestyle — that will translate into fat free and fit forever.

Here's a worthwhile hint: If you wear your Polar Heart Rate Monitor while you perform any of these activities, you'll be able to monitor yourself, making sure that you are maintaining your weight management zone — and burning the appropriate calories.

THE POLAR FAT FREE AND FIT FOREVER MAINTENANCE PROGRAM

Adding increased activity to your life is one way to maintain the changes you've recently made in your life. The Polar Program also recommends continuing to follow the 20-week program of the exercises of your choice. Simply use the "Maintenance" column on your chart or retest yourself and, using your Polar Heart Monitor, go for another fitness level at a higher target heart rate. I recommend you begin to increase your upper target heart rate by 5 percent at a time. For example, if you were exercising at 60 percent of your maximum heart rate, go for 65 percent — gradually building up to 70 percent. If you were exercising at 65 percent, go for 70 percent — gradually building to 75 percent. You can also maintain your new-found fitness by simply staying where you are: at a healthy point in the Weight Management or Aerobic Training Zone, exercising at least three times a week, and enjoying what you do.

The Polar nutrition program is just as easy to maintain. When you've reached a weight you're comfortable with, simply add zero to that number. Add your 200 "exercise" calories and you have your lifetime maintenance equation for lifelong good health and weight management!

Here's an example: Let's say you've reached your weight loss goal of 125 pounds. When you add your zero and your 200 "exercise" calories, you get a grand total of 1,450 calories a day — enough to maintain your goal and not feel deprived.

Exercise Exchange Lists

CATEGORY 1: OUTDOOR WORK*

1 AEROBIC EXCHANGE
(100 Calories)

Activity	Minutes of Activity Needed	
	Women	Men
Car		
Repairing	28	24
Wash and wax (by hand)	29	25
Chopping wood	16	13
Construction (general)	21	18
Gardening		
Digging	14	11
Hedging	22	19
Planting	16	13
Weeding	24	20
Mowing lawn		
Pushing hand mower	15	13
Pushing power mower	26	21
Painting house	22	19
Raking leaves	32	26
Shoveling snow	15	12
Stacking firewood	20	16
Sweeping	30	26
Window cleaning	29	25

---

*Calculations are based on 154-pound man and 128-pound woman. However, the heavier you are, the less time you will have to spend doing your activity to burn the calories you want. The lighter you are, the more time it will take to burn those calories.

To figure the calories burned subtract 10 percent from the minutes needed for every 15 pounds you are *over* the reference weight; add 10 percent to the minutes needed for every 15 pounds you are *under* the reference weight. For example:

It takes 32 minutes for a 128-pound woman to burn 100 calories raking leaves. Women A weighs 143 pounds.

Multiply $32 \times 10\%$: $32 \times .10 = 3.2$
Subtract 3.2 from 32: $32 - 3.2 = 28.8$

It would take Woman A approximately 29 minutes to burn 100 calories raking leaves.

It takes 26 minutes for a 154-pound man to burn 100 calories raking leaves. Man B weighs 139 pounds.

Multiply $26 \times 10\%$: $26 \times .10 = 2.6$
Subtract 2.6 from 32: $26 + 2.6 = 28.6$

It would take Man B approximately 29 minutes to burn 100 calories raking leaves.

Above calculation formula modified from *Physiological Fitness and Weight Control* by B. J. Sharkey. Mountain Press Publishing Company. Additional references can be found in the "Further Reading" section.

(The lists on the next 6 pages are taken from *The Exercise Exchange Program* by Dr. James M. Rippe, New York: Simon & Schuster, 1992)

CATEGORY 2: INDOOR WORK

1 AEROBIC EXCHANGE
(100 Calories)

Activity	Minutes of Activity Needed	
	Women	Men
Carpentry	22	17
Cleaning	28	25
Grocery shopping	28	25
Mopping floor	28	25
Musicianship (vigorous)	26	21
Painting walls	51	42
Plastering walls	22	18
Polishing furniture	52	43
Scraping paint from walls	27	23
Scrubbing floor	16	13
Standing (cashier/artist)	48	40
Stocking shelves	32	26
Sweeping floor	30	26
Tailoring	38	32
Vacuuming	38	30
Wall papering	36	30
Washing/drying clothes		
Automated	38	32
Hand washing small items	41	34
Hanging clothes to dry	29	25
Woodworking (light)	34	29

CATEGORY 3: LEISURE ACTIVITIES

1 AEROBIC EXCHANGE
(100 Calories)

Activity	Minutes of Activity Needed	
	Women	Men
Archery	26	22
Badminton	18	15
Billiards (shooting pool)	41	34
Bowling	34	29
Canoeing (slow)	39	32
Croquet	39	32
Cycling (5.5 mph)	27	22
(total miles)	(2.4 mi.)	(2.0 mi.)
Dancing		
Ballroom	34	28
Modern rock	10	9
Square or folk	15	13
Fishing	28	23
Hiking (no load)	14	12
Horse grooming	13	11
Horseback riding	23	19
Horseshoes	31	26
Ping-Pong	24	20
Rowing (slow)	24	20
Sailing	26	21
Scuba diving	8	7
Shuffleboard	34	29
Skating	15	12
Skiing (slow)	16	15
Sledding	17	14
Snowshoeing	10	9
Swimming (slow)	20	17
Water skiing	15	13

CATEGORY 4: RECREATIONAL SPORTS

1 AEROBIC EXCHANGE
(100 Calories)

Activity	Minutes of Activity Needed	
	Women	Men
Baseball (not pitcher)	25	21
Basketball	13	10
Boxing	10	8
Canoe racing	17	14
Cricket	20	16
Cycle racing	10	9
Fencing	11	10
Field hockey	13	11
Football (touch)	13	11
Golf (walking with hand-pulled cart for clubs)	20	17
Gymnastics	26	22
Handball		
Light/moderate	13	11
Vigorous	9	7
Horse Racing	13	10
Ice Hockey	13	11
Judo	9	7
Karate	9	8
Mountain Climbing		
(25-pound load)	12	10
Racquetball		
Light/moderate	13	11
Vigorous	10	8
Skiing		
Downhill, moderate	13	11
Downhill, racing	7	6
Rowing/crew racing	8	7
Soccer	13	11
Squash		
Light/moderate	13	11
Vigorous	8	7
Table tennis	25	21
Tennis		
Doubles	21	17
Singles	15	12
Volleyball	34	19

CATEGORY 5: CARDIOVASCULAR FITNESS

1 AEROBIC EXCHANGE
(100 Calories)

Activity	Minutes of Activity Needed	
	Women	Men
Aerobic dance		
Light-impact/moderate	17	14
Heavy-impact	13	11
Bench stepping		
11-inch bench, 18 steps/minute	20	16
11-inch bench, 30 steps/minute	12	10
16-inch bench, 18 steps/minute	15	13
16-inch bench, 30 steps/minute	9	8
Cycling (outdoor), 9.4 mph	17	14
(total miles)	(2.7 mi.)	(2.2 mi.)
Cycling (stationary bicycle ergometer, pedal speed 50–60 rpm)		
300 kgm (1.0 KP)	22	27
450 kgm (1.5 KP)	17	20
600 kgm (2.0 KP)	13	16
750 kgm (2.5 KP)	11	14
900 kgm (3.0 KP)	10	12
Cycling, Lifecycle—see Category 6		
Jumping rope		
70 jumps/minute	11	9
80 jumps/minute	10	9
125 jumps/minute	10	8
145 jumps/minute	9	7
Running		
Cross-country	11	9
12-minute mile (5 mph)	12	10
8-minute mile (7.5 mph)	8	7
6-minute mile (10 mph)	6	5
5-minute mile (12 mph)	5	4
Skiing, cross-country		
3 mph	13	11
(total miles)	(0.7 mi.)	(0.6 mi.)
8 mph	7	6
(total miles)	(0.9 mi.)	(0.8 mi.)
Stair climbing	17	14
Stair climbing, Lifestep—see Category 7		
Swimming		
20 yard/minute	26	21
(total yards)	(520 yd.)	(420 yd.)

CATEGORY 5: CARDIOVASCULAR FITNESS

1 AEROBIC EXCHANGE
(100 Calories)

Activity	Minutes of Activity Needed	
	Women	Men
25 yards/minute	20	17
(total yards)	(500 yd.)	(425 yd.)
50 yards/minute	9	8
(total yards)	(450 yd.)	(400 yd.)
Walking		
Track/treadmill		
3.0 mph	30	25
(total miles)	(1.5 mi.)	(1.3 mi.)
3.5 mph	26	21
(total miles)	(1.6 mi.)	(1.3 mi.)
4.0 mph	21	17
(total miles)	(1.4 mi.)	(1.2 mi.)
4.5 mph	16	14
(total miles)	(1.2 mi.)	(1.0 mi.)
Road, 3.5 mph	21	18
(total miles)	(1.3 mi.)	(1.1 mi.)
Field, 3.5 mph	17	14
(total miles)	(1.0 mi.)	(0.8 mi.)
Snow, 3.0 mph	8	7
(total miles)	(0.4 mi.)	(0.4 mi.)

YOUR POLAR HEART RATE MONITOR: A PERSONAL BODY WATCHER

Don't underestimate the value of your Polar Heart Rate Monitor as a weight management and fitness aid. It is the most reliable product in the world for guiding and monitoring your target heart rate, which is the key to effective exercise and weight loss. It can also help you watch your weight after you achieve your weight loss goal by taking the "guesswork" out of your exercise program.

Think of the Polar Heart Rate Monitor as your "Personal Body Watcher." It is the "window to your heart rate," which is the most accurate measurement of the cardiovascular fitness level of your body. Listen to your heart regularly as you exercise and it will help to keep you trim, fit, and healthy.

MAINTAINING MOTIVATION FOR MAXIMUM RESULTS

There are so many ways to keep motivation strong — and they can be as individual as the people involved. I know. I have talked to many people about their motivation, including those who have participated in our Polar study, others at the Exercise Physiology Lab and those who I have met in my years of experience as a cardiologist and fitness enthusiast. The number one motivational tool for many exercise "converts" was their Polar Heart Rate Monitor. It gave them immediate feedback; it gave them more purpose and even a sense of fun. Other tools varied from person to person. One individual changed her walking route from week to week so she wouldn't get bored and quit. Another person created interesting low-fat meals and set an elegant table to make dinnertime an "event." Another one charted her progress on a weight loss graph, seeing, in black and white, her weight loss "line" move down. Yet another person put a "fat" picture on her refrigerator — as a reminder to eat thin. Still another person set short-term goals that she could easily meet and feel good about; these included making sure she exercised three times a week, adding an extra half-mile to her walk, turning down a sugary dessert at a baby shower.

All these and more are suggestions to keep motivation high. In my experience, anything will work if it feels right to an individual. However, I have found the following seven tips to work quite well for long-term weight management and fitness:

■ **Tip #1: Make an appointment with yourself.** Most people find it easier to maintain their exercise program if they set aside a specific time to do it — instead of a casual "trying to fit it in" somewhere during the day that never works out.

■ **Tip #2: Ask for the support of family and friends.** If you let the people who are close to you know how important your weight and exercise program is to you, they will support your efforts. Maybe they'll even join you!

■ **Tip #3: Find exercises and foods you enjoy.** No one wants to continuously do something they hate — and I guarantee they won't do it for long. For success on the Polar Program, choose from our variety of exercises to find one you'll like. Pick food

Diet Plateaus

Any change involves periods of plateaus — and that includes weight management and improving aerobic capacity. There will be periods where your progress seems to have flattened out.

This is not true. The most important advice I can give you is don't panic. A plateau can simply be your body's way of consolidating the gains you have already achieved. If, however, a plateau has gone on for more than three weeks, I suggest trying a different Meal Plan; you may have inadvertently measured your food too generously. You might also try a longer workout or one at a sightly higher target heart rate.

The good news with plateaus is they don't last. Most likely you'll find a drop within a few weeks and the plateau will disappear.

exchanges that you find delicious; find some new, healthy meals to try in a low-fat cookbook.

■ **Tip #4: Use variation to prevent boredom.** Vary your walking or jogging route. Try a different workout tape. Pick a different breakfast instead of the usual cereal and milk. Try interesting grains such as kasha or couscous instead of the usual pasta and rice.

■ **Tip #5: Keep the risk of injury low.** There's nothing like pain to stop an exercise program in its tracks. The good news is that if you follow the Polar Program, you'll keep injury at an all-time low. But keep it up in the long run, too. Use your heart rate monitor as a "coach." Make sure you're not pushing yourself too much. Keep within your target heart rate zone.

■ **Tip #6: Avoid food "triggers."** Stress, emotional upsets, even good times can create diet havoc for the most motivated person. The best strategies include planning ahead for those "good times." This means saving your food exchanges for the party — or allowing yourself to enjoy it all and just exercise a little more the next day. On the other hand, emotional upsets can be better handled by some relaxation or deep breathing, even an indulgent bath. Remember, if you continue to eat all the wrong things, you'll have two problems: the emotional upset you started with and a weight gain. Another way to avoid "triggers": keep the foods you love most out of the house. Or, if you must give in, buy just one cookie or one scoop of ice cream from a bakery or soda shop — instead of purchasing a whole bag or pint container.

■ **Tip #7: Reward yourself.** Never, never forget yourself. You know how hard you've worked and you deserve a reward when you've reached even the smallest weight management goal. When you've lost five pounds or when you've exercised consistently three times in one week, reward yourself with some new music, tickets to a game, or even a night off with a video and a warm blanket. Reward yourself with anything that will make you feel good. Short-term rewards give you more motivation to achieve your long-term weight management and fitness goals.

•　•　•　•　•　•　•　•

Congratulations! You now have everything you need to make the Polar Fat Free and Fit Forever Program a success. I hope it will prove to be everything you want it to be. I know that the individuals in the Polar Fat Free and Fit Forever study lost weight, got fit, and felt great. I know that they were able to change their lives for the better.

It is my great wish that the information and tools you now have will promote weight management and good health in you. I hope that you will gain control of your life, of your day-to-day efforts. I hope that you will soon be on your way to a whole new way of life. A better one. A healthier one. And a happier one.

It can happen. The Polar Fat Free and Fit Forever Program will work for you.

Get started today!

I wish you well.

DR. JAMES M. RIPPE

APPENDIX A

The Different Types of Polar Heart Rate Monitors

Polar Electro Oy, the premier heart rate monitor company, offers its electronic fitness device in models tailored to the needs of people of all ages and fitness levels who want the safest and most precise way to lose weight and stay fit forever. The company produces five models: Polar Favor™, Polar Pacer™, Polar Edge™, Polar Accurex® II and Polar Vantage® XL.

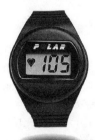

Polar Favor™

Polar Favor has a large 3/8" LCD that shows continuous heart rate. It is fully water resistant.

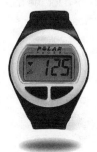

Polar Pacer™

A step-up model to the Polar Favor, this model offers target zone heart rate settings with alarms that signal to help you stay in your effective target heart rate exercise zone. It features a 1/2" LCD wrist watch display with time of day and alarm clock, and is water resistant.

Polar Edge™

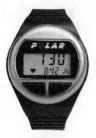

Designed for the fitness enthusiast, the Polar Edge features a dual LCD display which shows both continuous heart rate and total exercise time. It also features programmable hi-lo target heart rate settings and displays total time exercised above the lower limit. It is fully water resistant for swimming and also functions as a wrist watch with time of day and alarm clock.

Polar Accurex® II

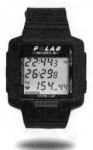

For the competitive athlete who wants the ultimate features for training and performance, the Polar Accurex II offers a triple LCD display with lap time, time-of-day, or stop watch and heart rate. The programmable hi-lo alarms can be set in single beat increments. Upon completion of your exercise, the Polar Accurex II displays average heart rate for the entire workout, and recalls up to 44 lap times with corresponding heart rates. It is fully water resistant to 20 meters and has complete sports watch functions with time of day, date and alarm clock.

Polar Vantage® XL

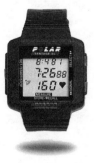

This premier model offers two sets of programmable target zone limits with alarms, stores up to eight separate workouts with more than 33 hours of information, and is computer compatible. It provides time of day with alarm, stopwatch, unlimited interval markers, two target zones and two workout timers. This model is intended for the more advanced fitness enthusiast, professional or elite athlete and for team use.

Hundreds of thousands of Polar's Heart Rate Monitors are in use throughout the world today. See your local Polar dealer for more information or call 1-800-227-1314.

Vital Statistics Chart

Name _____

Age _____ Date _____

	INITIAL TEST	10 WKS	20 WKS	CHANGE
BMI WEIGHT & CIRCUMFERENCES				
Weight	_____	_____	_____	_____
Waist (in.)	_____	_____	_____	_____
Abdomen (in.)	_____	_____	_____	_____
Buttocks (in.)	_____	_____	_____	_____
Mid Thigh (in.)	_____	_____	_____	_____
AEROBIC CAPACITY				
Heart rate, rest (bpm)	_____	_____	_____	_____
Heart rate, total	_____	_____	_____	_____
Test time *One Mile Fitness Walking Test* (bpm)	_____	_____	_____	_____

(Taken from *The Exercise Exchange Program* by Dr. James M. Rippe, New York: Simon & Schuster, 1992, p. 372)

APPENDIX C

The Step Fitness Test

(NOTE: Do warm-ups and stretches before you begin)

1. Find An Eight Inch Step

The easiest place to look may be the stairs in your home. If you decide to go with this option, measure your stairs to make sure that they're approximately eight inches in height. If your stairs don't measure eight inches, you may put together some sturdy boards and measure them to the approximate height.

2. Clothing

Dress in comfortable, loose fitting clothes and athletic shoes.

3. Taking The STEP Fit Test

The STEP Fit Test is a three-minute test conducted at a cadence of 76 counts per minute. It simply involves stepping up and down on the eight inch platform with a four count sequence as follows: right foot up on platform, left foot up on platform, right foot down on floor, left foot down on floor. Or, you may start with the left foot. Each time you move one of your feet, that is considered a count. For example, a four count sequence of up, up, down, down is considered four counts. You should accomplish 76 counts per minute.

A. Perform The STEP Fit Test by maintaining a cadence of 76 counts per minute for a period of 3 minutes. Try to keep a steady, comfortable pace. See part (B) below for more detail.

B. Here are three optional ways to time yourself for a 76 counts per minute cadence:

Use the second hand of your watch to assure that you complete approximately five of the four-count sequences in 15 seconds. (You may want to practice before taking the actual test.)

Or, set a metronome (as typically used for piano lessons) at a rate of 76 counts per minute, and move your feet one step every time the metronome clicks.

Or, call 1-900-646-STEP (1-900-646-7837) which will lead you through the entire test. The call is $3.95.

(Taken from *The Step Company Fitness Brochure*, Atlanta, Georgia: The Step Company, 1993)

C. At the end of three minutes, stop stepping and look at your heart rate monitor.

THE STEP FIT TEST RESULTS
How To Read Them And What They Mean

To find the results of your STEP Fit Test on the Relative Fitness Level chart, simply follow the steps below:

1. Find the Relative Fitness Levels charts for your age and sex.
2. Find your one minute heart rate (the one you took at the end of The STEP Fit Test) on the left side of the chart.
3. Lastly, the point on the chart where your Heart Rate and Activity Level meet gives you your fitness level as determined by American Heart Association standards. This is simply a way to compare your current fitness level with others of your same age and sex.

RELATIVE FITNESS LEVELS

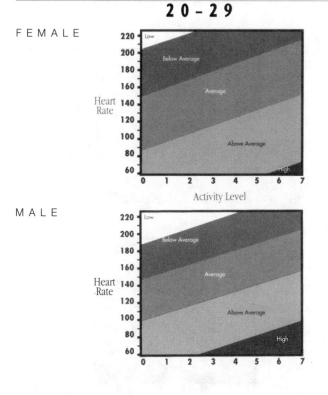

3 0 – 3 9

FEMALE

Heart Rate

Low
Below Average
Average
Above Average
High

Activity Level

MALE

Heart Rate

Low
Below Average
Average
Above Average
High

4 0 – 4 9

FEMALE

Heart Rate

Low
Below Average
Average
Above Average
High

Activity Level

MALE

Heart Rate

Low
Below Average
Average
Above Average
High

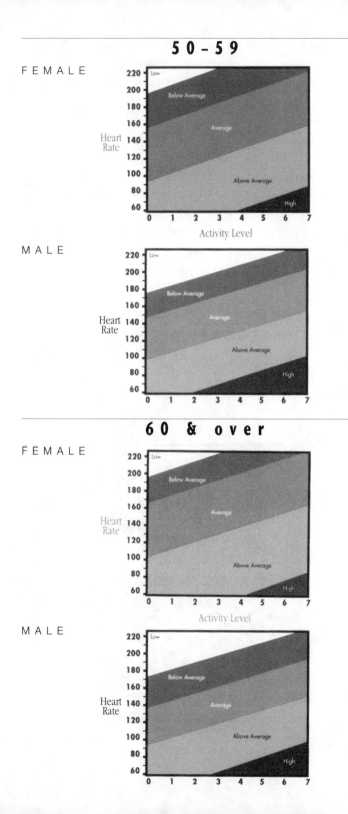

50 – 59

FEMALE

Heart Rate

Activity Level

MALE

Heart Rate

60 & over

FEMALE

Heart Rate

Activity Level

MALE

Heart Rate

1. Find the charts labeled *Fitness Stepping* Prescriptions. Find the one that corresponds to your sex and age, and mark the point where your heart rate and Current Physical Activity Level meet. This gives your personal *Fitness Stepping* Prescription — (A–blue, B–green, C–yellow, D–orange, E–red).

2. Now turn to the Fitness Stepping Program charts in Chapter Four. Find the program (A–blue, B–green, C–yellow, D–orange, E–red) that corresponds to your *Fitness Stepping* Prescription.

3. Start your *Fitness Stepping* Program and follow it for the next 10 weeks.

4. At the end of the 10 week program, take The STEP Fit Test again to determine your new aerobic fitness level and your next *Fitness Stepping* Prescription.

FITNESS STEPPING
PRESCRIPTIONS

20 – 29

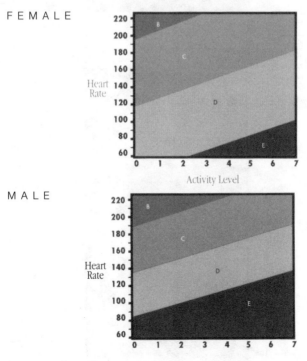

3 0 – 3 9

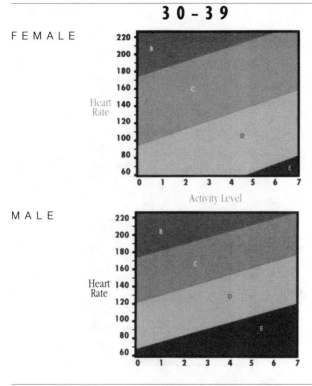

FEMALE

MALE

4 0 – 4 9

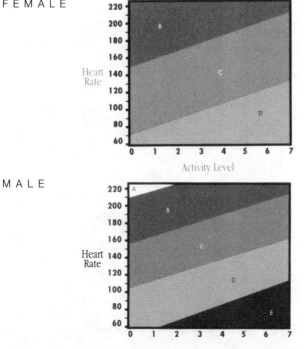

FEMALE

MALE

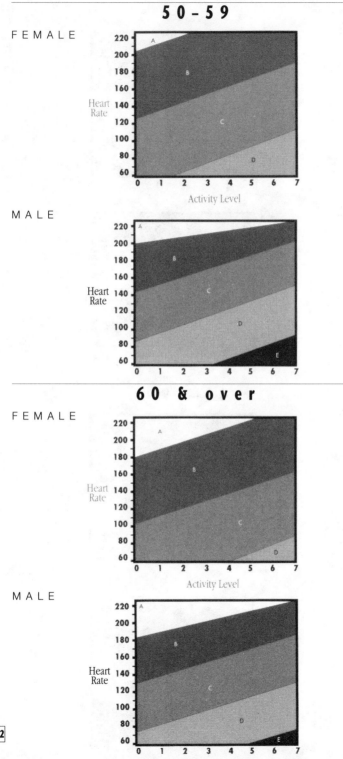

APPENDIX D

The Lifecycle FIT Fitness Test

In this program:

■ warm-up and stretch for five minutes before you start.

■ Then follow the directions on the Lifecycle console, which will guide you through the *Lifecycle FIT Test.*

■ Be sure to record that score on the vital statistics chart in Appendix B.

Now find the chart for your sex in this section and plot your score (also known as VO2MAX) against your age to determine your relative fitness level: very poor, poor, below average, average, above average, good, excellent, or elite.

Relative Fitness Classifications for Men

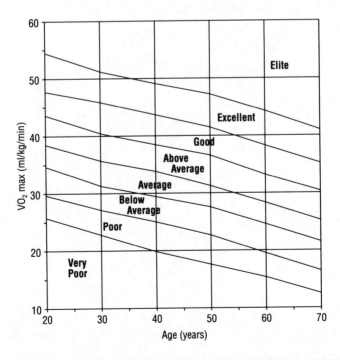

(Taken from *The Exercise Exchange Program* by Dr. James M. Rippe, New York: Simon & Schuster, 1992, pp.351-352)

Relative Fitness Classifications for Women

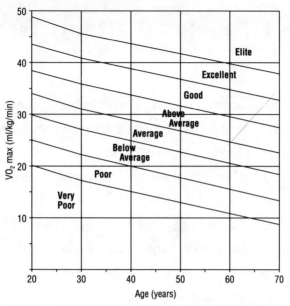

Then plot your score against your weight to determine the appropriate color group for your Lifecycle program.

Lifecycle Exercise Program

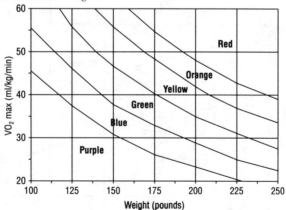

For example, if you are a 40-year-old man weighing 175 pounds whose FIT test score was 35, your relative fitness level would be above average (age vs. score). Your color for the Lifecycle program would be Green (score vs. weight).

APPENDIX E

A Blank Food Diary

Sample Meal Plan Menus

1,200-Calorie Meal Plan

4 MEAT	3 FRUIT
4 BREAD	3 FAT
3 VEGETABLE	2 MILK

80 OPEN CALORIES

BREAKFAST

1 orange
1 slice whole-wheat toast
1 teaspoon margarine
1 cup milk
coffee or tea (optional)

LUNCH

1/4 cup water-pack tuna mixed with
1 tablespoon reduced-calorie mayonnaise* on
2 cups garden salad
1 (1-ounce) whole-wheat roll
1 1/4 cup watermelon
1 cup milk

*Nonfat yogurt can be mixed in for a moister dressing

DINNER

3 ounces lightly sautéed chicken
1 baked potato, 3 oz.
1/2 cup cooked broccoli
1/2 cup summer squash
1 fresh peach or 1/2 cup water-pack canned peaches
noncaloric beverage

SNACK

3 cups plain popcorn with 1 teaspoon margarine
noncaloric beverage

OPEN CALORIE SUGGESTIONS:
Increase toast at breakfast to 2 slices, or add a medium apple for a snack, or add 1/2 cup low-fat frozen yogurt for dessert at dinner.

(Taken from *The Exercise Exchange Program* by Dr. James M. Rippe, New York: Simon & Schuster, 1992, pp.38-40)

1,500-Calorie Meal Plan

5 MEAT	4 FRUIT
5 BREAD	3 FAT
3 VEGETABLE	2 MILK

200 OPEN CALORIES

BREAKFAST

1 orange
2 slices whole-wheat toast
1 teaspoon margarine
1 cup milk
coffee or tea (optional)

LUNCH

1/2 cup water-pack tuna mixed with
1 tablespoon reduced-calorie mayonnaise* on
2 cups garden salad
1 (1-ounce) whole-wheat roll
1 1/4 cup watermelon
1 cup milk

*Nonfat yogurt can be mixed in for a moister dressing

SNACK

1 small pear
noncaloric beverage

DINNER

3 ounces lightly sautéed chicken
1 baked potato, 3 oz.
1/2 cup cooked broccoli
1/2 cup summer squash
1 fresh peach or 1/2 cup water-pack canned peaches
noncaloric beverage

SNACK

3 cups plain popcorn with 1 teaspoon margarine
noncaloric beverage

OPEN CALORIE SUGGESTIONS:

Add 1/2 tablespoon jelly at breakfast, add 1 ounce string or low-fat cheese to the afternoon snack, and increase potatoes at dinner to 2 servings.

1,800-Calorie Meal Plan

6 MEAT	4 FRUIT
6 BREAD	4 FAT
4 VEGETABLE	2 MILK

300 OPEN CALORIES

BREAKFAST

1 orange
2 slices whole-wheat toast
1/2 tablespoon (1 pat) margarine
1 cup milk
coffee or tea (optional)

LUNCH

1/2 cup water-pack tuna mixed with
1 tablespoon reduced-calorie mayonnaise* on
2 cups garden salad
1 (1-ounce) whole-wheat roll
1 1/4 cup watermelon
1 cup milk

*Nonfat yogurt can be mixed in for a moister dressing

SNACK

1 small pear
noncaloric beverage

DINNER

1 tomato, sliced
4 ounces lightly sautéed chicken
1 baked potato, 6 oz.
1/2 cup cooked broccoli
1/2 cup summer squash
1 fresh peach or 1/2 cup water-pack canned peaches
noncaloric beverage

SNACK

3 cups plain popcorn with 1 teaspoon margarine
noncaloric beverage

OPEN CALORIE SUGGESTIONS:

Add 1 tablespoon jelly at breakfast, omit roll at lunch and add 2 slices rye bread for a tuna sandwich, add 1 ounce string or low-fat cheese to the afternoon snack, and increase popcorn to 5 cups, and increase margarine to 2 teaspoons at the evening snack.

APPENDIX G

Pocket-Sized
Target Heart Rate Zone
and Meal Plan Exchanges

Side One:

> **My Weight Management Zone range is _____ to _____**
>
> **My Aerobic Training Zone range is _____ to _____**

Side Two:

	Fruit	Milk	Meat	Bread	Vegetables	Fat	Open
1,200	3	2	4	4	3	3	80
1,500	4	2	5	5	3	3	200
1,800	4	2	6	6	4	4	300

SOURCES

Cachero, A.J., "The Effects of Feedback on the Maintenance of Exercise Heart Rate in the Target Training Zone." Columbia University Program in Physical Therapy Thesis, May 1991.

Carlucci, D. Goldfine, H., Ward, A., Taylor, P., Rippe, J.M., "Exercise: Not Just for the Healthy Part II: The Health Benefits of Exercise." *Phys and Sports Med 19(#7):46*, 1991.

Ebbeling, C.B., Ebbeling, C.J., Ward, A., and Rippe, J.M., "Comparison Between Palpated Heart Rates and Heart Rates Observed Using the Polar Favor Heart Rate Monitor During an Aerobics Exercise Class," Exercise Physiology and Nutrition Laboratory, University of Massachusetts Medical School, Worcester, MA, December 1991.

Edwards, S., *The Heart Rate Monitor Book*. Port Washington, New York: Polar Electro, OY, 1992.

Fletcher, G.F., et.al.: "AHA Medical/Scientific Statement on Exercise: A statement for health professionals by the committee on exercise and cardiac rehabilitation of the council on clinical cardiology." American Heart Association, 1992.

Freedson, P.S., Ward, A., Rippe, J.M., "Childhood health and fitness." *Encyclopedia Britannica Medical and Health Annual*, 1990.

Goldfine, H., Carlucci, D., Ward, A., Taylor, P., Rippe, J.M., "Exercising to Health: What's Really in It for Your Patients? Part I: The Health Benefits of Exercise." *Phys and Sports Med 19(#6):81*, 1991

Kashiwa, A., Rippe, J.M., *Rockport's Fitness Walking for Women*. New York: Perigee Books, 1987.

Lissner, L., Odell, P.M., D'Agostino, R.B., Stokes, J. III, Kreger, B.E., Belanger, A.J., Brownell, K.D., "Variability of body weight and health outcomes in the Framington population." *N Engl J Med 324:1839-1844*, 1991.

Rippe, J.M., Ward, A., Porcari, J., Freedson, P.S., "Walking for health and fitness." *JAMA 259:2720*, 1988.

Taylor, P., Ward, A., Rippe, J.M., "Exercising to Health: How Much, How Soon? Part III." *Phys and Sports Med 19(#8):95*, 1991.

Taylor, P., Ward, A., Rippe, J.M., "How to Tailor an Exercise Program. Part IV." *Phys and Sports Med 19(#9):64*, 1991.